HAPPY
GENETICS

RICHARD ROMAGNOLI
PIER MARIO BIAVA

HAPPY GENETICS

FROM EPIGENETICS TO HAPPINESS

Selectbooks, Inc.
New York, New York

This edition published by SelectBooks, Inc.
For information address SelectBooks, Inc., New York, New York.

First Edition
ISBN 978-1-59079-510-1

Library of Congress Cataloging-in-Publication Data

Names: Romagnoli, Richard, author. | Biava, Pier Mario, author.
Title: Happy genetics : from epigenetics to happiness / Richard Romagnoli, Pier Mario Biava.
Description: First english edition. | New York, New York : Selectbooks, Inc., 2021. | Includes bibliographical references and index. | Summary: "Authors combine findings in the modern sciences of epigenetics and stem cell research with practices of ancient wisdom to advocate a path to reverse illness and stress. They believe by simply choosing laughter, happiness, and love as the driving force for change and following healthy daily routines we can restore the balance of body, mind, and emotions-- Provided by publisher".
Identifiers: LCCN 2020050109 (print) | LCCN 2020050110 (ebook) | ISBN 9781590795101 (paperback) | ISBN 9781590795149 (ebook)
Subjects: LCSH: Happiness. | Laughter. | Love. | Mind and body. | Epigenetics.
Classification: LCC BF575.H27 R663 2021 (print) | LCC BF575.H27 (ebook) | DDC 158--dc23
LC record available at https://lccn.loc.gov/2020050109
LC ebook record available at https://lccn.loc.gov/2020050110

Art direction for the original Italian edition by Davide Cortesi

Manufactured in the United States of America
10 9 8 7 6 5 4 3 2 1

To Loretta Zanuccoli
for having poured the wisdom
of love into this world

CONTENTS

HAPPY

FOREWORD

"Impossibility is only a whole of greater possibilities not yet realized."

These words by the great Indian philosopher Sri Aurobindo came to my mind several times while reading the passionate research path that Doctor Pier Mario Biava tells us about in these pages.

That's the way it really goes: the obstacles and difficulties that suddenly interpose between us and our goals can forcefully distance us from the established path but, precisely for this reason, they can also evolve into unexpected turns, creative solutions, real discoveries.

That happens particularly when a person comes to a state of balance. In fact, whoever is in self-awareness never looks at things from a single point of view, but is open to seeing, listening, and interpreting all the stimuli. Then the mind often succeeds in detaching itself from the mechanisms of linear thought—the one linked to the cause-effect criterion that characterizes the Western world—to access speculations that tend to proceed in a circular sense. Therefore, the conclusions are often overturned with respect to the premises, and continually modify them.

It is precisely in this way that the impossible became a reality for Pier Mario because he did not surrender before the first results, because he kept an open mind, because, as he himself writes, he remained faithful to his dreams.

We are talking about scientific research, of course, but also about research in an intensely human sense.

And it is precisely this aspect that strikes us from the first pages of the book with the warm story overflowing with gratitude for its origins, returning in vivid images of a childhood immersed in a melancholy, muffled atmosphere. A dimension that could also have led to an isolation to the bitter end, had instead inspired an acute capacity for introspection and the most tenacious aptitude to believe in one's dreams emerging from a fertile soil of self-awareness.

This process is not dissimilar to the journey deep within ourselves when we find ourselves face-to-face with the disease and decide to undertake a way to dissolve conflicts of the soul that often become conflicts of the body—a journey that leads us to question all that we are and can make the disease itself an opportunity for evolution and growth.

In fact, during this expedition to the roots of our essence, we may find ourselves discovering that the path taken crosses many other branches: the path of the heart, the path of gratitude, that of joy, and finally that of forgiveness. Forgiveness of others but also, and above all, of ourselves.

Every path we decide to walk amplifies our ability to listen to our most intimate inner vibration and to tune into it more and more in a progressive and growing revelation. The extraordinary discovery that all around us is vibration, everything is life, and each of us is connected to everything and everyone.

This is an important book because it speaks to us of the need for today's medicine to open up to new scientific paradigms and to finally look at the human being in its totality: mind, emotions, body and spirit, past and present history, inner and outer conflicts, dreams, expectations, relationships, and social connections.

Nevertheless one who says all this in these pages is not a mystic, a philosopher, a poet or a psychologist, but a scientist accustomed to dealing with both the solidity of extremely concrete data, and with the extraordinary results already obtained. And this is what gives even more strength and resonance to his words.

In fact, I am increasingly convinced that the real re-evolution for humanity will be the convergence—in various fields of knowledge—of two apparently opposite points of view. In this case I am speaking on one hand of the point of view of those who have always explored the nature of human interiority, and on the other hand the point of view of scientists, those who are traditionally concerned with clarifying the nature of the object and of the world. And this desirable synergy will have wonderful implications on countless aspects of life for each one of us.

The rigorous scientific research of a scientist like Pier Mario Biava and the insights and irresistible laughter of Richard Romagnoli, an expert on Laughter Therapy methodologies, are a splendid example of this kind of harmonious convergence. Both, in fact, consider with great attention—and total absence of separation or duality—the complexity of the energies, emotions, and experiences that, in the long run, can affect the mechanisms of our body and manifest themselves as physical discomfort.

Laughter Therapy, which Richard has generously committed to spread throughout the world, allows pranayama, the ancient art of breathing, to be practiced naturally. At the same time, with Laughter Therapy we benefit from the well-being that is propagated at a physiological level while we learn to laugh for a long time and, so to speak, with the whole body.

This body of ours, which has its own intelligence, and which we should respect as a temple, deserves our reverence. But because we are distracted we have no awareness of it. We have lost the ability to listen because we are not present. Therefore, unfortunately, in the world in which we live the body is no longer the "temple of the soul." Instead, it is often treated as a hedonistic object that we try to forcefully shape into its form, into a program that has little to do with a true healthy balance and, not infrequently, hides a subtle death anxiety.

Love, on the other hand, is the key, as is also claimed in these pages. Love is the amazing "molecule" giving to each one of us the ability to perform miracles and transform life—our own and that of those around us—into a continuous propagation of positive energy that, like ripples on water, extends to infinity around us.

Love, beauty, gratitude, and joy are the fire, the energy that can fuel our every action, our every experience. This is why a happy mood contributes greatly to creating, or recreating, the harmonious balance of our body.

However, it is not a question of hiding wounds, of denying the suffering of the soul or the body. On the contrary, as in the ancient Japanese art of *kintsugi*, which uses gold instead of transparent glue to fix a cracked vase, it is a question of dealing with painful experiences as a peculiar part of existence that precisely for this reason makes every person unique and precious.

We Westerners, however, have serious difficulties in relating to cracks, break-ups, fractures in our souls and our bodies. It happens because the mechanistic thinking trains us to see only one aspect of reality: something is intact or broken.

Then, in the delicate symbolic message of kintsugi we can identify a true teaching for us to learn the art of embracing our painful experiences to come to terms with them by reopening an authentic channel of communication.

Similarly, today science tells us that in the face of diseased cells, a bombardment of chemotherapy is not the only way forward.

We can also try to give back to the cells that original information which, evidently, had been lost. Exactly the same way, in life and in the world of work, one can try to understand what was misunderstood at a certain point in the relationship and thus try to re-establish the communication that had been broken.

And here, in the continuous osmotic flow of life, dichotomies and opposites cease to be such. Then, the "breaking" of an object, but also of a relationship or an internal organ, does not necessarily represent its end. Life, in fact, is at the same time integrity and rupture; it is constant and eternal recomposition.

In this regard, I find deeply moving the increasingly evident parallelism between the assertions of contemporary physicists and the timeless intuitions of the mystics: relativity, interconnection, and non-permanence.

Today science tells us that in the spectrum of reality everything is matter, energy, and information at the same time. There is information within everything: atoms, cells, stones, human beings, plant forms. And it is precisely information that moves life and allows it to manifest itself.

The universe is ordered by different energies in continuous balance. However, it is not one energy against another, but harmony full of love, some wise intelligence. Love: this invisible conscious intelligence that moves everything.

Niccolò Branca

HAPPY

"The happiest people
are not necessarily
those who have the best of everything,
but those who make the best
of what they have."

KHALIL GIBRAN

1

BE ALWAYS HAPPY

RICHARD ROMAGNOLI

Dad clasped my hands tightly and looking into my eyes told me: *"Be always happy."* My heart started beating wildly, and I managed to respond with a whisper: *"I promise you, Dad."*

That evening, in the hospital room where he had been lying for some time, I fell asleep thinking about his words, the last ones he told me before leaving his body. For many months he had struggled with a terrible disease, which had struck him when I was still a boy. I can proudly say I loved Dad so much. I admired him for his ability to be loved by many people beyond his friends and family. I admired his ability to inspire colleagues with his dedication to his work, and I was in awe of his great generosity and the joy of life that was an innate gift that enabled him to draw smiles from even the grumpiest people.

Dad had the ability to transform the grayest days, making them suddenly beautiful, like those rainbows that suddenly appear after a storm and hover lightly towards infinity.

In the last period of his illness I promised myself to find a way to alleviate the suffering of those in pain. I could not understand how medical science, despite the many wonderful breakthroughs, could still be so inadequate and unable to effectively find the right treatments for cancer patients like him. For a long time Father had subjected himself with great confidence to all the therapies recommended by the doctors. I remember the continuous operations he underwent due to the seriousness of the illness and the endless days spent with him in the hospital trying to distract him and comfort him during the suffocating sessions of radiotherapy and chemotherapy. During this experience, I was able to observe that it is precisely in moments of discouragement that those who suffer find in the smiles and words of encouragement of doctors and paramedics the strength they needed, which relieved them from at least some of their suffering.

I have a sense of enormous respect and profound gratitude to all those who practice the medical art, who recognize the importance of the necessary therapeutic alliance established between doctors and the patients under their care that has been so wisely declared by two luminaries, Edmund D. Pellegrino and David C. Thomasma.

At such a gloomy time, in which I went through long weeks full of anguish, I tried in every way to soothe my inner suffering. I felt powerless in the face of Dad's suffering, and the only thing that remained for me to do was to turn to God to ask him the reason for all that experience. I wanted to know, from his point of view, what was the use of all that pain, demanding a full answer from the Creator himself.

It is in moments of difficulty that our faith strengthens or weakens. Even those who do not place faith in any creed, and who experience moments of intense pain, feel the need to re-establish intimate contact with their inner serenity so that the mind can quiet itself down. During that difficult time I suffered more because of the lack of mental serenity. It was as if my peace of mind had been completely engulfed by the anger and profound disappointment I felt. I only began to emerge from that deep darkness when I resumed my studies on Eastern spirituality. After Dad left the body, I began to think seriously about dedicating myself to the study of medicine. I felt the need to deepen my knowledge of all the scientific topics concerning the body-mind bond. I hoped to find the answers to the many existential questions that had remained buried and unresolved in me. In my heart I longed to become the doctor that Dad should have met, and that could explain the reason for his illness, helping him to heal deep inside.

I was certain that in order to understand human nature and to alleviate our suffering, I would have to study human beings in their entirety. Like a loner who embarks on an unknown journey, I began to venture out, exploring knowledge and the subtle links that connect body-mind-emotions-soul as one.

Traveling to discover unknown destinations is fascinating, as is the very mystery of the unknown. To proceed towards knowledge it is necessary not to be influenced by the limits of what is already known, it is necessary to be willing to have that open mind, which allows us to be surprised by new knowledge, which can emerge only beyond preconceptions and mental limits.

Today, unlike the past centuries and thanks to modern scientific experiments, we recognize that the human being can no longer be considered as a simple compound of chemistry and molecules or as a set of organs and apparatuses that interact with each other mechanically. We are aware of the fact that our real identity cannot be illusory and confused with our gross body, which is nothing more than an essential tool that allows us to live the experiences of life, to experience and discover our true and real Divine Nature.

One day I made a choice, and it was that instead of dedicating myself to the study of medicine, I would dedicate myself to exploring another knowledge, the most intangible—and perhaps for this reason—the most fascinating: the science of the Soul.

I began to deepen the studies I had already undertaken at sixteen on various topics concerning spirituality, this time round with more commitment. Re-reading the Vedas I began to reflect on the various teachings of my beloved Master Sri Sathya Sai Baba with a different perspective. I felt the need and a sense of urgency to reach conclusions that would help me make Peace with God. Rather than needlessly wasting time following sterile philosophical dissertations, I began the most adventurous of journeys, the introspective one.

It so happened that in search for the lost meaning of what had happened to me, in an unconventional and somewhat bizarre way I began to practice well-being, with the Soul as the starting point.

THE MAGIC OF LIFE

My passion for the art of prestidigitation gave me the opportunity to embark on a wonderful adventure, without which I could never have lived through all the experiences that over the years have allowed me to meet thousands and thousands of people around the world, and even in large audiences to make them experience the therapeutic power of unconditional laughter.

By dedicating myself to voluntary service in hospitals, I began to recover from the trauma and the pain of losing my father. It all happened when I accepted the invitation to perform in a small provincial hospital.

My experience in hospital wards led me to the understanding of how a positive attitude is important and necessary, both for hospitalized patients and for the relationship between operators and doctors in healthcare facilities.

When I was eight, Dad managed to get special permission from the board of the psychiatric hospital where he worked for me to perform before their in-patients. After my magic show an old lady came up to me and hugged me.

Her tender gesture dissolved all my fears, and that day, in that psychiatric hospital, I decided that one day I would dedicate myself to doing something that would bring relief to the lives of the most marginalized people. I was only eight years old, and that very day I unknowingly sowed a powerful seed in my destiny, which today I cultivate with joy.

In everything we do, what really makes a difference, and sets us apart, is the intensity and the love with which we do it. This applies to our family and professional lives, as well as to the rapport between those who experience the disease and those who must take care of them. We often focus more on operational routines or on what needs to be done, rather than on the person receiving care. Simple gestures like a smile, a hug, a caress, as well as words of comfort, have the great power of bringing about positive change to people's lives.

We must begin to understand that every gesture of love remains indelibly impressed in those to whom we give it.

IT WILL BE ALL RIGHT

When Sara and I decided to move to southern India for a long stay, it was to carry on with the volunteer service in hospitals and orphanages in the Indian subcontinent, which I had already started a few years earlier. With our girls Matilde and Sofia we moved to Puttaparthi, one of the poorest states of India, but really rich in spirituality.

Our Master had proved to be benevolent toward us regarding that drastic decision to leave Italy forever and to change our Western habits and adapt ourselves to learning local customs.

I have always believed that when choices are made with love and awareness, the subsequent consequences always bring the best in one's life. A few years after our move to India, our beloved Master left the physical body, and after a few months of loss due to that experience, my mission continued with more fervor than before pursuing a single goal, that of contributing to well-being of the greatest number of people in the world or, more simply, of being at the service of humanity.

With more diligence than before, I continued to attend Sri Sathya Sai Super Specialty Hospital in Puttaparthi, doing my volunteer service and receiving endless gifts, thanks to the unexpected learning opportunities that enriched my life with new teachings.

I found myself attending the best doctors in India. I was following a select group of professors and luminaries of various medical specializations with whom I volunteered thanks to the Sathya Sai Mobile Hospital project.

Every month, for twelve consecutive days, the Mobile Hospital carries out an incredible humanitarian service for which it has been honored with world-wide praise, bringing to different Indian villages every kind of care necessary for the thousands of unprivileged people who otherwise would not be able to afford all the treatments necessary for their cure because of their poverty.

The Mobile Hospital is equipped with the most sophisticated medical equipment and allows thousands of children, women, and the elderly to be visited by the best professors and doctors who spend their holidays devoting their time to this voluntary service with a spirit of devotion.

In those months I learned the importance of heart-to-heart communication that allowed me to interact with the children and the elderly of the villages even though I did not know their local languages. To bring them some relief my contribution was to entertain them by trying in every way to encourage smiles and unleash their laughter. Being with those doctors allowed me to learn more than what is taught in many university programs. Observing their attitudes and studying their ability to empathize with older people, women, and children has revealed to me everything that can never be learned by studying from textbooks. Knowing how to listen is ninety-nine percent the secret of effective communication because it allows us to establish, with greater success, the real needs of those who are in front of us. From those doctors I learned how fundamental it is never to forget that every cure, every drug, and every relationship that is established with those who are sick must have a single purpose: their well-being.

One day walking along the main street of Puttaparthi I received an unexpected gift, which I have described in my first book *I Learned to Laugh.*" I entered a small bazaar and bought a small book that allowed me to discover that in Mumbai, India in 1995, an Indian doctor had started a revolutionary movement, and a methodology that included the union of yogic and meditation practices, with laughter exercises to promote the well-being in people. The ancient Indian scriptures, the yoga masters and the sages have always reminded the Indian people of the importance of happiness and joy, which were intended as devotional practices necessary to succeed in spiritual disciplines. In India Hasya Yoga, or the yoga of laughter, has ancient roots and has been practiced for centuries as a yogic and ascetic practice. The ones who laugh are defined as wise because they remain unaffected by the effects of Maya, by the phenomenal illusion of this creation, for in their state of awareness they do not feel attachment to the ups and downs of life, and are free from all feelings and suffering.

The purchase of that book was certainly not accidental. It was a moment of serendipity, which put me in connection with my destiny. As I read further, I realized that I was receiving an answer to the request I had made several months before, in the presence of my Master, when I had asked him to let me find a technique or methodology, a philosophy or any other useful knowledge to help the greatest number of people in the world to rediscover inner happiness. Finally after several months I had found what I was intuitively looking for.

When I met the Mumbai doctor whose book I had read, he had just moved a few hours from Puttaparthi, on the outskirts of Bangalore. I attended one of his courses and five days later I became a teacher of his amusing methodology. Back home I put into practice the techniques I had learned, and so every morning at five, instead of practicing the other techniques I had learned during my studies in India, I practiced laughter meditation. Experimenting on myself with the cathartic and therapeutic power of laughter, and the benefits related to greater oxygenation of the body, I decided to open the laughter club in Puttaparthi at Saraswathi Hall.

This marked the beginning of an experience that then allowed me to travel the world spreading the methodology of unconditional laughter everywhere, in schools right up to universities, hospitals and companies, and to train hundreds and hundreds of trainers who today in different countries in the world continue to spread the teachings received, helping people to break down stress by laughing and relaxing deeply. Back in Italy, thanks to the experiences and knowledge learned in India, and above all thanks to what I received from my Spiritual Master, my teaching began to spread irrepressibly from north to south, expanding beyond European borders. To date I have met hundreds of thousands of people to whom I have been able to donate the best of what I have learned, and above all experienced. To think that all this happened thanks to a moment of serendipity! It makes me smile at my Master with deep gratitude.

One day I had a private meeting with Devi Amma, the wise Indian woman who lives in Whitefield. She talked to me about my future and reassured me by saying these simple words: "*It will be all right.*"

I have always believed in Amma's words because love never lies, and it is what animates the truth.

"THERE ARE MANY ROADS THAT LEAD TO THE DIVINE;
I HAVE CHOSEN SINGING, DANCING, AND LAUGHTER."

—*Rumi*

HAPPY

"One must be happy
around the sick."

THERESE OF LISIEUX

2
YOU ARE NOT YOUR DISEASE

RICHARD ROMAGNOLI

When people identify with their disease, they become victims of a misperception moving away from their real identity. We live a life completely dedicated to carrying out what we have to do; we are increasingly busy acting, suffocating that primordial impulse that allows us to discover our true existential nature. Too much importance has been given to the body rather than actually considering it for what it is—a vehicle—the means through which we experience this earthly existence, made of joys and sorrows, of contrasts and continuous alternations.

Any action taken becomes important when it is based on the awareness of who we are.

If we confuse our reality with what we appear or think we are, we deny the beauty, wisdom, and inner knowledge of which we are custodians and confessors.

There's more to us than what we think we are. In a small seed it is enclosed everything that will make it, in time, a wonderful plant. Imagine if the seed thought it was not destined to become that plant: it would limit itself to be what it isn't.

It often happens that we are the first ones who cannot recognize our true inner potential; it is as if we were that dormant seed, unable to recognize its natural essence. Starting to appreciate us more for what we are, we begin to rely on our inner strength and to reveal our essence through the experiences of our life.

When I was 12, I asked myself: "Who am I?"

I remember writing right away on a sheet of paper all the answers I could think of. Several years later I went to India for the first time to meet my Master. One day Baba approached me, smiled and asked me: *"Where do you come from?"* I immediately said: *"From Italy, Swami."* He gave me a puzzled look, as if my answer was wrong or incomplete and started to walk away slowly, leaving me in doubt about what I had just answered. In the following months, after returning to Italy, I asked myself again about the reason for his question, and I tried to guess the best answer I should have given him.

A couple of years went by, and I finally returned to India to my Master. One day Baba recognized me among thousands of his devotees, and when he came over to meet me, he asked me: *"Where do you come from?"* Looking at him straight in the eye my heart started beating like crazy, I thought I shouldn't get it wrong, and so I remained silent, contemplating him. At that moment I felt that the only thing I could do was to admire his sweet and compassionate gaze; then silently I informed him of the answer I had in my heart. Normally when someone asks us where we come from, we say what our city is or our country of origin, but when it is a Spiritual Master who asks us this question, its meaning changes because he is leading us to a much deeper level of understanding, which is not a mental, but an existential one. That day, finding myself in the presence of the Master, the most authentic answer that sprang from the silence of my mind was the one coming from the voice of my heart. The Masters and sages who have experienced their existential nature are aware that they are beyond their body, beyond their mind, recognizing that they are part of a whole.

BEYOND BODY AND MIND—THE SELF

The great Spiritual Master Sri Nisargadatta Maharaji used to say: *"When you realize that the destination is the road and that you are always on the road, not to reach a destination, but to enjoy its beauty and its wisdom, then life ceases to be a duty and becomes simple and natural, a blessing in and of itself."*

If for a moment we recognize ourselves for what we are, getting rid of the limited perception we have of ourselves, we will find we can go beyond all the limits we have imposed. By starting to investigate the nature of the mind, we begin to discover how much the physical, psychological, and emotional well-being are closely related to its functions, as neuroscience states.

Unfortunately, we have allowed our mind to make us slaves of impulses and sensory desires, remaining subdued by continuous and uncontrollable thoughts, fantasies, and useless desires, so that instead of improving the quality of our life, we stray from the true sense of ourselves.

It is necessary to find out how we can make best use of the features of our mind, so that it is at our service and not vice versa, in order to understand who we are, what is the nature of life, and what is the purpose of our existence. By totally identifying ourselves with the senses and the body we effectively limit our real nature, trivializing our very existence. It is as if we identify ourselves with the car we are riding in, ignoring the fact that we are the passengers. If we own a car we need to keep it in good condition, doing the maintenance, occasionally checking oil levels and making sure of the proper functioning of brakes, tires, and engine. Likewise we can consider our body as a special vehicle that we must maintain in good condition through proper physical training and proper nutrition and striving to cultivate a harmonic approach between mind, psyche, and emotions. Sri Sathya Sai Baba often recalled: *"The body is the vehicle for the journey of life. If the vehicle is not properly maintained, we should be ready to deal with serious problems on the way."*

The body is an immense gift, entrusted to us for a limited time, and our responsibility is to take care of it. We all know that those who abuse harmful substances, those who smoke and those who excessively drink alcohol, severely damage their own bodies, thus putting themselves at risk of serious diseases. In order to avoid repercussions, it is necessary to act on these weakening and negative habits and to replace them with new, happy, and positive ones. We are responsible for the health of our body, and it is necessary to understand that stress, that we create and foster on a daily basis because of wrong life habits, is one of the main causes of the onset of psychological problems and mental illness, gastrointestinal and skeletal-muscular disorders, and other diseases.

Analyzing the quality of the life we lead, both at work and at home, we realize the frantic pace we are subjected to and how unsustainable and counterproductive this is for the maintenance of a balanced physical, mental, psychic, and emotional well-being. To escape stress is a complex matter, but if we take a pause to reflect on what our real needs are, we can determine how to regain possession of the appropriate amount of time to engage in activities we enjoy, and this will enhance our mental and physical well-being. Why should we cause ourselves discomfort and disease? Compared to the past centuries, thanks to the extraordinary discoveries of medical science and neuroscience, we now have the possibility to prevent many of the known diseases by adopting more healthy eating and life habits. With an increased awareness of our lifestyle based on respect toward ourselves and all other existing forms of life, we can do a lot to improve our fate and nourish hope for a life which is as healthy and complementary to our nature as possible.

"NEVER MOVE YOUR SOUL WITHOUT YOUR BODY,
NOR THE BODY WITHOUT THE SOUL, SO THAT DEFENDING EACH
OTHER, THESE TWO PARTS MAINTAIN THEIR BALANCE
AND THEIR HEALTH."
—*Plato*

EMPATHY: THE LANGUAGE OF HEALING

According to a scientific study published a few years ago in the magazine *Annals of Human Biology*, the cells that make up the human body are more than thirty-seven thousand billion, and if we think that the Milky Way is composed of "only" two hundred billion stars, we can consider our body a well-organized cosmos.

As we know, the skeleton consists of over two hundred bones, while the muscles of an adult human body are over seven hundred and the organs seventy-six. The current scientific research, facilitated by the use of increasingly sophisticated technological instruments, demonstrates the marvelous complexity of our body, which is a real laboratory, multifunctional and highly specialized. If we disregard all the already known definitions that have been used to better define our body-mind complex but begin to approach with interest the most recent scientific discoveries, such as those provided by quantum physics, it becomes clear how limiting it is to think of "our body" without recognizing it as being part of a manifestation infinitely more vast than we know.

After going through dark historical periods of the evolution of humanity, today we have reached a crossroad when consciously or unconsciously each of us decrees through our daily choices the future of the planet and the fate of humanity. We are all connected into a single large multidimensional network of subtle energies which, in addition to feeding human beings, feeds the life of more than 8.7 million varieties of living species. When most of the world's population will be aware of the principle of unity that drives it and of the fact that each of us belongs to one great world brotherhood, then we will witness a deep change that will allow wars to cease, and the gradual disappearance of those disturbing elements that continue to violate the peace, security, and well-being of peoples and nations.

Those who incite violence and trigger wars or those who think to enrich themselves by taking advantage of other people's weakness, ignore the fact that they will be the first ones to suffer the consequences of the cosmic law of cause and effect. As we begin to know ourselves better, we will evolve to a new inner dialogue in our rational mind that will lead us straight to our spiritual heart to that epicenter where all our existential answers are based. No remedy is really as effective as the awareness of who we are and of the extraordinary strength which comes from our balanced mental attitude.

⁓⁓

THE SELF THOUGHT:
"HOW CAN ALL THIS BE WITHOUT ME?
IF SPEECH IS MADE BY THE TONGUE, BREATH BY LUNGS,
SIGHT BY EYES, HEARING BY EARS,
SMELL BY THE NOSE AND MEDITATION BY THE MIND,
THEN, WHO AM I?"
—*Aitareya Upanishad*

⁓⁓

As Professor Biava has already widely explained, when a body gets sick, there are different triggering factors that cause cellular degeneration and disturb its metabolic balance.

While fundamental treatments allow the body to regain its balance, it is equally necessary that sick people are helped to restore their mental and emotional harmony. When we begin to study the various energetic-vibrational aspects that interact with the body, we begin to recognize the impact that our thoughts, words, and actions have on our life style and therefore on the ability to maintain a good physical, mental, and emotional health. The importance of the physician when communicating the diagnosis to the patient is widely demonstrated. It is necessary for the doctor to know how to create a correct and balanced empathic contact with the patient and his family. Why should a sick person who addresses doctors with confidence be psychologically destabilized because of incorrect communication by those who are responsible for protecting their health? Why should a caring language not be adopted in hospital environments, where care, kindness, and hospitality are most needed? Why should a patient be considered a number to be registered rather than a human being to be treated and lovingly cared for? When a diagnosis is communicated to the patient with an attitude of deep respect, it is precisely in that moment that a strong trusting relationship is established, which is necessary to those who must be cared for and those who will take care of them. The doctor should always be at the patient's service and never the other way round. Every day hundreds of thousands of health care professionals carry out a delicate mission, offering their humanity and professionalism at the service of those who need their care.

ഇ൦ ഇ൦

"DOCTORS MUST INSTILL COURAGE IN PATIENTS
AND TALK TO THEM QUIETLY,
RADIATING COMPASSION AND LOVE.
THE APPROACH THUS ESTABLISHED HAS A GREATER INFLUENCE
ON RECOVERY OF PATIENTS THAN PRESCRIBED MEDICINES."
—*Sri Sathya Sai Baba*

ഇ൦ ഇ൦

Words spoken with warmth and attention are a soothing balm for the mind. People remember long afterwards the exact words spoken by doctors when they were talking about their diagnosis. The disease, in addition to being evidence of a functional imbalance, represents the need of those who experience it to regain a better quality of life and to determine to have a more peaceful management of their relationship with themselves during their illness.

If medicine was only a huge business, no one could really take care of those who suffer, because patients would become the unaware customers of a deal called disease.

There is a process that transforms every patient into a consumer when the doctor prescribes medicines to the patient, who trustingly buys them in a pharmacy. Pharmaceutical companies, as we know, produce these products called medicines and restock shelves of pharmacies through their distributors. If people were healthier, an economic system that has existed for decades would collapse because fewer medicines would be sold, causing a serious collapse of the global economic and financial system.

According to the most recent statistics, the trend of consumers of medicines is increasing, and it is expected that in the coming years, with the increase of the aging of the world population, the consumption of chemicals will increase and this will inevitably benefit the revenues of the pharmaceutical multinational companies. Only when the prescription of drugs aims at relieving the suffering of patients, and they are administered for therapeutic reasons or for curative or preventive purposes, and when this is in a logical pursuit of the real welfare of the people in respect to ethics and universal human values will this be basically lawful. But when interest in sick people is primarily aimed at its speculation and is lucrative, then "Big Pharma" proves to be one of the greatest failures of humankind.

The responsibility of pharmaceutical companies and that of scientific researchers and doctors is truly enormous, and it must be more recognized by governments that must be the guarantors of the rights of citizens, not the protectors of lobbyists. For this reason, it is necessary that those who directly or indirectly are involved in the great mission of being at the service of the sick, are aware that the only logic to follow and protect is one that points to the well-being of the people, in order to restore balance to a system that has been eroded on many levels from the serious corruption of our health services that has been so detrimental to our world.

Respect for the patient and adequate attention to their needs should always be exercised by professional health workers as well as the patients' families. Establishing ethical and caring relationships with ill people who are going through difficult and traumatic experiences has a considerable effect on their recovery and return to well-being.

There are many aspects that need to be taken into account and that can help the patient to get back in shape. By stimulating and experiencing positive emotions our body is able to produce in a more relevant way the chemicals that are intended for its healing.

In the early 1980s clown therapy was accredited by hospitals. The practice of smiling was observed to be important to improve patients' moods and supported the efficacy of humor therapy to enhance psychological treatments of patients. Already in the seventeenth century in Italy, the Carmelite priest Angelo Paoli, who was beatified in 2010, loved disguising himself to bring a little bit of hilarity and relief to the sick and especially to children; he is considered one of the forerunners of the clown therapy. This was then brought into the spotlight by Karen Ridd in Canada and by Michael Christensen, the "father of pediatric clown care" in the US. Later Hunter "Patch" Adams made clown therapy famous in American hospitals and all over the world.

Today pet therapy, which was born in the sixties thanks to the intuition of the child psychiatrist Boris Levinson, is recognized in hospitals as a care practice in support of therapies, in virtue of the special relationship that grows between patients and pets.

In recent decades thousands of scientific research studies have demonstrated and validated the importance of beneficial practices such as mindfulness, and more recently of the effectiveness of unconditional laughter for the psychophysical improvement and recovery of patients. Numerous research studies carried out in the field of neuroscience have credited medication for being one of the most effective wellness practices on several levels: physical, emotional, and psychological.

⌒⊙◡⊙⌒

"HEALTH IS A STATE OF COMPLETE PHYSICAL,
MENTAL AND SOCIAL WELL-BEING,
AND NOT MERELY THE ABSENCE OF DISEASE OR INFIRMITY."
—*World Health Organization, 1948*

⌒⊙◡⊙⌒

When the body is suffering from a disease, we call the person "sick." But that person is not the disease. If in the winter when we happen to catch the flu we say: "I have the flu," not "I am the flu." However, in Italian for instance, people often express themselves using phrases to the effect of: "I am colded" or "I am flued" without realizing that this way of expressing themselves demonstrates an ambiguity in their mind about what has happened to their body.

In his masterpiece *In Search of Lost Time* Marcel Proust wrote: *"The pathogenic agent, which is a thousand times more virulent than all the microbes, is the idea of being sick."* When you suffer from a disease the fact is not immediately recognized that it is a part of the body suffering from that disease, because our ego easily identifies itself, both psychologically and emotionally, with the disease itself. Our personal beliefs influence the concretization of reality even before it manifests itself. In addition to providing the necessary care for your recovery, it is often necessary to heal the very idea that you have of being sick. Healing must be considered not only from the physical point of view, but on multiple levels that are interdependent among themselves and that make up a whole: Body-Mind-Emotions-Soul.

How is it possible to treat a stress-induced gastrointestinal discomfort without taking into account the underlying cause? The purpose of every cure is not to treat the effect, but to extinguish the cause.

If the alarm that is installed in our house goes off, what will be our concern? To turn off the alarm or to find out if there are intruders inside our house? And if we find out that there are thieves inside, what do we do? Do we turn off the burglar alarm or do we act to restore order and security within our home?

In the same way, when our body is sick, it begins to inform us, just as it happens with the burglar alarm, of some malfunction or an imbalance or of the presence of some 'intruder' inside itself and, therefore, of the need to act with a specific intervention to restore balance in the physiological and biological functions of the body. The disease informs us, allowing us to act on its cause.

"In humans, in particular, it was concluded that
there is no dualism between mind and body,
but that the organism works as a single cognitive
network in which the genome constitutes
the code of signification."
—*Professor Pier Mario Biava*

WHAT SCIENCE CANNOT REACH, THE WISDOM OF LOVE CAN

Research in the field of neuroscience have shown that traumatic events are a contributing factor to the onset of diseases and related mental disorders, which in medical jargon are defined post-traumatic stress disorders.

The cells follow the complex information they are equipped with to perform their functions. We may imagine them as equipped with a GPS navigator, capable of providing them with all the detailed information in order to follow a well-defined path and to act in accordance with their assigned role. As soon as the cells, due to certain factors, lose contact and communication with the navigator, missing their original way, they confuse their role, coming into conflict with that of the other cells. This gives rise to a malfunction in the system, resulting in a traffic that is not controlled and irregular and that can lead to accidents of variable seriousness, which subsequently we shall call disease.

Approaching the knowledge that regulates complex cellular systems is extremely fascinating, but it is also easy to get lost in the maze of a research that seems to have no boundaries and that leads researchers further and further away from their own insights.

❧ ❧

"THE MOST IMPORTANT THING IN MEDICINE?
IT IS NOT SO MUCH THE DISEASE FROM WHICH THE PATIENT
SUFFERS AS THE PERSON SUFFERING FROM THAT DISEASE."
—*Hippocrates*

❧ ❧

I often asked myself: Is it possible to know the unknowable? Will it be possible for science to determine infinity in the near future? If today you can explore the three-dimensional structures of biological molecules with the use of advanced cryo-electron microscopes, what will happen in the near future when the evolution of nano-technologies allow researchers to use instruments that are inconceivable today? But already today there is a thousand-year-old science within reach that offers us the possibility to investigate where no microscope or nanotechnology will ever gain access, and this is what is known as the science of the Soul.

Like other sciences, inner investigation also deserves to be recognized for its importance in our lives. Spiritual philosophers and researchers have always posed important existential questions in the hope of being able to provide appropriate answers to the meaning of life. As the applied sciences study in detail the functioning of each single part of the body and human behavior, so the science of the Soul illuminates us about how to reach our most intimate part, our true reality, also called Truth.

One of the scientists of inner research was Saint Augustine of Hippo who wrote: *Man cannot understand the way in which the spirit is united to the body, and yet in this union constitutes man.*

An Augustinian monk, the famous Gregor Mendel, was the forerunner of modern genetics, and it is thanks to his studies and observations on hereditary characteristics that research was begun which today is being carried on by contemporary scientists.

The science of the Soul transcends every other science because the exploratory investigation leads beyond the mind, going beyond all that is objective and subjective, without using the multisensory qualities our body is endowed with to perceive, explore, observe, and experience our reality.

The science of the soul leads us back to our essence, while the other sciences have the purpose of giving proven explanations on the functional, biological, psychological, and other kinds of mechanisms.

In order to discover the marvel of the human body we have to study its anatomy; to know and to deepen the functioning of the brain we have the studies and researches of neuroscience; to investigate the workings of the human mind, we can use psychology. But if we really want to know ourselves and give a meaningful answer to the question "Who Am I?" then we can do so only trusting our inner knowing, to which we can have access only if we can accompany the mind to the door of our interior laboratory. In this regard, one day Sri Sathya Sai Baba, during a public speech that he gave in 1992, said:

Some identify themselves with their body, not realizing that the body is transient and may disappear at any moment like an air bubble in the water.

Death will take those who identify with their body by surprise. The elements that constitute the body are five: ether, air, fire, water and earth, and it is corruptible; while the Being, who dwells within, is permanent, has neither birth nor death, and is, indeed, the Divine itself. The man who considers himself as an ephemeral body wastes his life. There are others who are misled and waste their lives by identifying with their minds. They are people who torment themselves with thoughts and fantasies, they whine about the past and make conjectures about the future; so they neglect the present and are always in a state of confusion. Then there is a third category of people for whom rationality is of the utmost importance, they identify with their own intellect, use it and embark on various projects. However, by exalting the virtues of Reason, they end up disregarding their true nature, which is divine. Therefore, the divine potential of the intellect itself is wasted and a life is spent in endless research and experiments. No matter how much research and investigation can be carried out, reason will never serve to understand the Divine. A fourth category of people has placed all their trust in the power of the antah-karana, that is, the internal organ of action, which includes mind, ego and intellect.

They seek to fulfill the Divine by taking the spiritual path, because they consider the phenomenal world as separate from them. The fifth category is the one of the man who says: "I am everything; there is nothing separate from me in the world." He is aware of the unreality of the world and has understood the Prâjña principle relating to the ego, that is, he is in a constant and integral divine awareness. In order to make body, mind, intellect and antahkarana be one and to identify the trascendental aim, we need to go beyond the mind, the intellect and the antahkarana and overcome the states of waking, dreaming and deep sleep. Only then will it be possible to understand the principle of divine awareness, or Prâjña. Body, mind, intellect and the antahkarana are related to the phenomena of nature, and are functional variants of the mind. God cannot be understood through thought and the mind should be kept under control with every effort.

HAPPY

"Love is the ultimate meaning
of everything around us.
It is not a mere sentiment; it is truth;
it is the joy that
is at the root of all creation."

RABINDRANATH TAGORE

3

LOVE IS EVERYTHING AND CAN DO ANYTHING

Love is our true essence. From the moment of our conception, love manifests itself as a powerful energy that allows our body to form and our consciousness to know itself, to explore itself. Love has no form; it is beyond time and every other circumstance. Love is everything and can do everything, and in order to appear, it must be able to flow freely over the mental barriers and the obstacles of desire, of attachment, doubt, and judgment. Love is an indefinable energy, which escapes the understanding of all sciences and which has always motivated psychologists and psychoanalysts to study its mechanisms—that is, those which guide human beings to make certain choices in relation to others. Why does a mother sacrifice herself during the months of pregnancy? What makes a man jump into a river to save a drowning child? And what motivates a firefighter to save an old man from a devastating fire? The answer to all these questions goes beyond the very sense of duty, and I believe that the real motivation, the one that allows each one of us to do the best for our good and for the good of our loved ones and society and nature, is to be sought only in love.

Love is that inexhaustible source that over the centuries has inspired artists, poets, musicians, and philosophers to compose works and poems, to make sculptures and paintings to communicate and inspire us to the beauty. In different ages, Spiritual Teachers, with the example of their lives, have inspired mankind to love, revealing to us their knowledge and inspiring us to practice in order to manifest our spiritual Self and to recognize the DNA of our soul.

Every day, according to the many interactions that we establish with others, we mix our love with an indescribable variety of other feelings that color and give life to new experiences and to new emotional nuance. I have always considered love as the art of living, of which we are artists and spectators. The ancient Greeks divided love into four forms: the first was "storge," the love for family members; "philia" was affection for friends; "eros" described the passion and attraction between two human beings, while "agape" defined pure love of a spiritual nature. According to psychology, love is a relationship between two people based on an emotional exchange, which responds to the psychological needs of affective exchanges and to the physiological need of sexual gratification. If we analyze love from a philosophical point of view, we could indefinitely debate this issue that is also the backbone of the major religious traditions.

One day it naturally came to me to ask which religion God belonged to, and it was by chance that as I read the words of my Spiritual Teacher, I found an authentic and exhaustive answer:

"There is only one religion: the religion of Love. There is only one caste: the caste of humanity. There is only one language: the language of the heart. There is only one God and he is all-pervasive."

Love motivates and influences our choices and pushes us to act to satisfy its impulses. For some people, the need to be loved is predominant, rather than to love. For others, unselfish love is part of their own lives, and to make a selfless service for the well-being of the community and the preservation of nature is a real mission.

There is much confusion with regard to love, so much so that what we can feel towards ourselves is often confused as an act of selfishness.

In fact, we can define selfishness as everything we do solely for ourselves with the primary goal to satisfy our personal needs, even if this proves to be to the detriment of the welfare of others. Excessive personal interest can result in mental pathology because the most selfish people are the saddest, those who suffer from loneliness because of the lack of authentic interpersonal relationships. The egotists are those who consider themselves better than others and who believe themselves to be the depositories of sublime qualities, talents, and high knowledge. Those who suffer from egotism have an exaggerated narcissistic consideration of themselves and this causes a deep psychological and emotional imbalance in them. People who have a high self-opinion think they are worth more than others, but in reality their social behavior is altered compared to reflect what they really are.

Is it possible to recognize what selfish actions are compared to those that are not? All the times that we choose to undertake initiatives that benefit our physical and mental health, these actions will have a positive impact on all those with whom we come in contact, first of all our family members. We often find great excuses not to act because we do not believe we have time to give to ourselves or because we prefer to sacrifice it to our family. Come to think of it, every week we have over a hundred and sixty hours, and if we fail to get at least an hour to ourselves, this happens for a simple reason: we are not able to optimize the time we have at our disposal. There is absolutely nothing wrong with considering our health important by taking care of it. If we really think we do not have time to dedicate to ourselves, we are renouncing something important to a piece of our happiness because no one else can take care of our own well-being better than us. If there was a scientific rule, which could expand and multiply happiness in every corner of the planet, this would be a simple but irrefutable formula: "Be the first one to be happy, to be able to make all the others happy."

Starting to dedicate the right time to ourselves to get more in tune with our well-being by encouraging and amplifying feelings of peace, serenity, harmony, and love. The well-being we will generate in our lives will spread in all our relational areas, including work.

According to statistics carried out by observers dealing with prevention and health in a professional environment, workers who at the end of the day feel strongly stressed and deprived of their vital energy are constantly increasing. The World Health Organization (WHO) expected that in 2020 depression would be the greatest cause of the inability to work. Many factors cause the spread of stress in people's relationships with their family and at their workplace. I believe that in addition to taking ordinary and perhaps extraordinary measures determined by law to help people on a social level, it is also essential for individuals to protect their own physical, mental, and emotional well-being.

Each of us has the duty to change this negative trend that is spreading like a true plague on society. To improve our life, it is necessary to restore a balanced and loving relationship with ourselves. Learning to loosen and unload the tensions accumulated during the day allows us to re-appropriate not only our serenity, but also our time and quality of our affective relationships, normally undermined due to this deficit of care towards us.

"YOU CAN SEARCH THROUGHOUT THE ENTIRE UNIVERSE
FOR SOMEONE WHO IS MORE DESERVING OF YOUR LOVE
AND AFFECTION THAN YOU ARE YOURSELF,
AND THAT PERSON IS NOT TO BE FOUND ANYWHERE.
YOU, YOURSELF, AS MUCH AS ANYBODY IN THE ENTIRE
UNIVERSE, DESERVE YOUR LOVE AND AFFECTION."

—*Buddha*

Love is a positive attitude toward oneself. When we act to improve our character, touching up our ego and polishing it with the tools of patience, love, and forgiveness, we can be certain that our inner work will bring out, more and more clearly, our best parts that may otherwise remain buried in the debris of fear, shame, resentment or any other negative feeling.

We very often fail in self-love because we are in conflict with ourselves. We think we cannot accept all those events that have marked the history of our lives to transform them into wisdom. Instead of accepting ourselves, we prefer to flee from ourselves by taking care of and caring for everything that helps keep us away from our personal growth. Instead of welcoming the new experiences of life, we become obsessed with the fear of the future and renounce instead of welcoming the best of life, which is there and ready for us to take if only we let it find us.

During my professional experience I have had the good fortune to meet thousands of people, and the ones that more than others enriched me inwardly were those who through their choices were able to prove themselves despite the severity of the drama they lived, because of their steadfast faith and trust in themselves and in life. Thanks to their strength of mind and their ability to be resilient to despair at the injustices suffered, they demonstrate by their example how important it is never to succumb to the fears created by the mind, but to feel more love towards themselves by choosing with courage and confidence to take back their lives and recapture, step-by-step, their space and happiness.

How much does it cost in terms of energy to choose to be happy, despite everything? Never trying costs a lot more. Why should we retreat or surrender to the ghosts of fear and anger rather than deciding to turn events into our favor by changing our way of interpreting them? The most extraordinary people, those who deserve the Nobel Peace Prize because they consistently nourish the world with harmony, are those who have chosen to be happy rather than succumbing to the negativity of life. But what motivates these people to be so happy? Love.

Love for themselves and love for their loved ones, friends, nature, and their ideals and human values. Because love is everything and can do everything.

"WHEN ILLNESS ATTACKS YOU, YOU ARE YOURSELF THE CAUSE,
BECAUSE YOU HAVE INTERIORLY NURTURED DISORDER:
YOU HAVE NOURISHED CERTAIN THOUGHTS AND FEELINGS,
YOU HAVE MANIFESTED CERTAIN ATTITUDES
THAT HAVE AFFECTED YOUR HEALTH.
THE BEST WEAPON AGAINST THIS DISEASE IS HARMONY:
DAY AND NIGHT TRY TO SYNCHRONIZE,
TO PUT YOURSELF IN ACCORDANCE, IN CONSONANCE WITH LIFE."
—*Omraam Aivanhov*

Some time ago I met a lady, who after undergoing yet another surgery, decided to realize one of the greatest dreams of her life: to go around the world in the company of her beloved dog. The lady told me that thanks to the experiences she enjoyed with people of different cultures, she managed to restore the inner harmony that she had lost. Love is the best cure that helps to prevent discomfort, that is, the difficulties that manifest themselves because of its lack. Out of love for themselves, people learn to act protecting their physical and mental health to prevent inconveniences and absolutely avoidable diseases. Each year millions of Euros are allocated for the prevention of various diseases and, thanks to monitoring programs and assistance plans for citizens, these important checkups allow us to safeguard our most valuable asset, our health.

Caring for one's physical body, as well as caring for one's mental and emotional health, is a duty for which we all need to take responsibility. During my training courses I always ask people how much time they devote to themselves, and the answer I generally get is "little time." Why? Because we are mentally and physically engaged elsewhere, and when we can have some free time to dedicate to ourselves, we waste it worrying about irrelevant things rather than investing it in our well-being. Today more than ever we need to consider as a priority the time to devote to ourselves in order to best nourish our lives. If love is the cure, we can all heal ourselves, manifesting this extraordinary energy in our relationships that comes from ourselves.

Love should, without any doubt, be the modus operandi of those professionals who work every day for the well-being of people. During a public speech, Sri Sathya Sai Baba said: *The greater disease is the lack of peace; when mind finds peace, body finds health, and therefore, those who yearn for a good health, must pay attention to the emotions, feelings and motives that animate them. As you wash your clothes regularly, you must wash dust and slag out of your mind; otherwise if dirt accumulates and creates habits, it becomes difficult to get rid of stains, as well as it is damaging to your clothes. Therefore the washing process must be daily: you must be careful that mud is not deposited in your mind! This is like saying that you must join a company that avoids dirt; falsehood, injustice, indiscipline, cruelty and hatred form filth, while Truth, Righteousness, Peace and Love are detergents. If you inhale the pure air of virtue, your mind will be free from evil viruses and you will have a strong mind and a strong body.*

To love oneself is to recognize that we are part of a wonderful whole, experiencing that joy that expands when we recognize that we belong to the whole planet Earth and its wonderful creatures. The divisions, conflicts, and all the thoughts that feed hatred and rivalry arise in the mind and, because of the attention given to the mind, we continue to experience in our life feelings of duality that take us away from our Divine Nature.

If we were to be asked to change the mental attitude of someone in our family with whom we had a disagreement, or that of any of our colleagues, we would be aware of accepting a challenge of uncertain outcome; but if we were asked to change our mental attitude, thanks to a greater knowledge and awareness of ourselves, we definitely would have more chances to succeed. Each of us is the true managing director of the actions of his own life, and once we are aware of the power we have towards ourselves, we can live a more fulfilling, peaceful and harmonious life.

When we recognize the fact that thoughts convey the mental energy, we can improve the quality of our physical, mental, emotional, and spiritual well-being through our introspection, simply by acting and making choices that are consistent with our human values.

The awareness of having this extraordinary energy available to us, that is conveyed through our thoughts and manifests itself concretely through actions, allows each of us to recognize himself as the depositary of the universal force, the same that nourishes our own life.

Each of us, every single moment of our existence, can choose to take action thanks to the awareness of love, the irresistible force that in addition to motivating us is actually our real essence— the cause and effect of every event, both tangible and intangible, known and unknown.

⤖⤗

"LOVE IS THE MASTER KEY
THAT OPENS THE GATES OF HAPPINESS."
—*Oliver Wendell Holmes*

⤖⤗

HAPPY

"To be happy, one must be free,
and to be free, one must stop accumulating
burdens on one's shoulders.
Joy is associated with the idea of lightness;
and what makes us light?
Love.
Joy is one of the most
poetic expressions of Love."

OMRAAM MIKHAËL AÏVANOV

4

THE JOY EFFECT

RICHARD ROMAGNOLI

Experiencing happiness is the right antidote to unhappiness. When we are cheerful we feel that our mood is great and our positive mental attitude predisposes us to react rather than succumbing passively to the duties and challenges of everyday life. When I was a little boy, Mike Buongiorno on TV greeted viewers with a big energy blast, rejoicing with his joyous: "Allegria!"

The expression "Heaven helps happy people" is based on the fact that happiness is mainly a state of mind we nurture in ourselves to induce our well-being, allowing us to attract the best from our life experiences. In some situations, remaining cheerful throughout the day can be a real challenge, especially when life puts your personal peace severely to the test, but you need to be aware of the truth that Albert Einstein proclaimed when he argued that no problem can be solved while maintaining the same level of consciousness that created it.

William James, enlightened American psychologist and philosopher, wrote: "The most important finding of my generation is that man can change his life simply by changing his own mental attitude." If we want to change anything in our lives, it is good go to the roots of the problem rather than circumvent the obstacle and get lost in its multiple effects.

If we want to change our mental attitude to pass from a negative state to a positive one, we can take action by making a change to our physiology, causing our body to experience a state of high well-being thanks to the production of the "happiness chemical," the one our body is perfectly capable of producing by positively influencing our psyche. When we listen to good music, when we dedicate ourselves to physical activity, when we spend time in good company by taking a walk in the open air, or when we choose to eat wholesome foods that nourish our body in a healthy way, we foster in ourselves the production of many chemical substances that are a real panacea for our health. When the mind is serene our mental attitude is totally different from those times when we feel stressed, agitated, and restless, and it is for this reason that daily practices such as mindfulness, meditation, and other practices of happiness, such as unconditional laughter, are necessary to help our mind regain harmony and balance. Often we are too busy highlighting problems and divisions and criticizing others, rather than stimulating the correct vision and rejoicing in our daily goals. Because of the bad habit of focusing on everything that is not right, we often forget our enormous good fortune to have received all the things that contributed to the well-being of our lives. Remembering the gifts received and those who took care of us allows us to experience at multiple levels a powerful healing energy and gratitude. Being grateful toward those who love us, those who work with us, and those we meet along our journey, we are able to produce a powerful vibration of love that creates harmony between thought, word, and action. My Teacher urged us to consider the importance of the three H's to have a life of true wellness, that is, the coherence between Head, Heart, and Hands. When head is connected to heart, man is able to make gestures that become a valuable contribution to the well-being of humanity.

Those who act in the world by separating their head from their heart selfishly take advantage of others, trampling on others because they are ignorant of the principles of fair conduct and lack fundamental values of truth, peace, love, and nonviolence. They create continual disharmony in their own and other's lives, making every experience on earth a real hell.

LAUGHING IS BREATHING. BREATHING IS LIVING. SO LAUGHING IS LIVING.

Considering how the world is going on, it is necessary for each of us to be the proponent of a positive change, the one that cannot be delegated to anyone else. It is necessary to make ourselves immune to the energy that creates the prevailing pessimism that is a grey cloud above our head preventing us from admiring the light and colors of life.

If we look at the dynamics of the mind we can understand that it often tends to project us to what happened in a more remote dimension of time. Rather than relive the rewarding experiences of our past, our attention is focused on the most difficult and painful events that we had to live, causing the risk of reigniting in ourselves all those negative feelings of anxiety, sadness, and repulsion that we have already experienced in the past. If we look at the dynamics of the game of life, we are able to assess how problems and difficulties have been the messengers of important teaching for our evolution, because their primary purpose is to make us aware that we must emancipate ourselves from the negative emotions that have given rise to our conflicts and unhappiness.

Through the writing of this book, Professor Biava and I want to share with as many people as possible who are sensitive to the topics discussed in *Happy Genetics*, the urgent need to encourage a profound change in our society to recover harmony and well-being and restore enthusiasm and happiness in the lives of as many people as possible in the world. We are aware that there are millions of human beings in the world who are ready to act to restore the balance in our fate on Planet Earth, because there is no economic, political, or religious power that can take possession of our awareness. Within the next few years, we will find what has already begun: our awareness that we can overturn the selfishness and nepotism of those who have written a sad chapter in the history of humanity.

"YOUR VISION WILL BECOME CLEAR
ONLY WHEN YOU CAN LOOK INTO YOUR HEART.
WHO LOOKS OUTSIDE, DREAMS.
WHO LOOKS INSIDE, AWAKES."
—*Carl Gustav Jung*

In 2016, when I established the Guinness World Record for the longest marathon of laughter therapy in the world that lasted twenty-four hours and thirteen minutes in a row, I was able to experience how the energy of unconditional laughter is extraordinarily powerful and able to evoke a multitude of latent energies. You do not need to set world records to benefit from this cocktail of happiness, that chemical that is released in our body when we laugh, because it is sufficient to laugh for a few consecutive minutes, or even better if we can do it often during the day to benefit immediately from a positive body and mood change.

Numerous scientific research studies published in the most prestigious and important international medical journals have shown for several years that laughter stimulates our brain to produce certain chemicals that are considered critical for the well-being. Thebeta-endorphins, for example, are protein hormones that serve as neurotransmitters and have a positive impact on our mood, allowing us to improve our psychophysical resilience to both negative stress and to fatigue and pain. Laughing inhibits the production of cortisol, the stress hormone, and increases the production of serotonin, called the hormone of happiness because the activity of serotonergic neurons improves the mood.

Laughter helps to relieve inflammation by reducing the formation of thrombus, thanks to the dilation effect of blood vessels, allowing an improvement in the circulatory flow. Other studies on the therapeutic effects of laughter have shown that when laughing, there is an increase in the activity of immune cells called NK lymphocytes (natural killer), which are useful to combat different types of diseases.

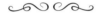

"WE DON'T LAUGH BECAUSE WE'RE HAPPY,
WE'RE HAPPY BECAUSE WE LAUGH."
—*William James*

In India, laughter is considered to be the equal of other important yogic pranayama practices, the ancient science of the yoga of breath, because laughing stimulates rapid and rhythmic contractions of the diaphragm muscle fibers, producing a massage of the abdominal organs, which in turn stimulate the digestive and liver secretions. When we laugh we exhale a greater amount of carbon dioxide than when we breathe normally. This allows us to empty our lungs of residual air and to rake in a greater supply of oxygen, essential for cellular metabolism as well as for tissue oxygenation and all the physiological functions. I have already written in my previous books on the importance of laughter as a daily practice of well-being, and

I can assure you that when laughing becomes a happy habit there is a profound change in the life style of people.

What would happen if doctors told their patients to laugh at least three times a day? First of all, there would be less pouting people, but above all many fewer sick people to take care of, as the administration in large doses of happiness, cheerfulness, and joyfulness keeps away diseases such as depression. Who has ever seen someone rejoice in happiness and be depressed at the same time? Who knows why laughter is so often stigmatized in school environments when students need to express their joy of living and learning. Maria Montessori said: *To teach you need to excite. However, most people still think that if you have fun, you don't learn.* Professor Roberto Assagioli, psychiatrist and founder of psychosynthesis, recalled the importance of laughter and smiling in the school environments for the development of students intelligence: "We should teach everything in order to make the pupil laugh, because laughter has a general and constant quality which is very important from the psychological side, that is the powerful, safe and lively excitement of attention. In fact, one of the main difficulties of the teacher is to make the pupil pay attention, to interest him in what he is taught."

Laughter has an indescribable power, especially in removing those heavy invisible boulders that are created by emotions such as fear, anger, or resentment.

⁘

"IN ORDER TO ACHIEVE THE STATE OF INNER FREEDOM
IT IS VERY USEFUL TO USE HUMOR ESPECIALLY TOWARDS YOURSELF:
TO MAKE FUN OF OUR PERSONAL LITTLE SELF SO FULL OF ITSELF,
WHICH TAKES ITSELF SO SERIOUSLY AND IS SO SENSITIVE!"
—*Roberto Assagioli*

⁘

In a study conducted by a group of American researchers headed by Professor Lee Berk and published in the international scientific journal *The Official Journal of the Federation of American Societies for Experimental Biology,* it has been highlighted that laughing in a sustained manner produces the same positive effects that Tibetan Buddhist monks experience in meditation by virtue of the stimulation of the gamma waves which, in that state, vary from 31 to 40 Hz.

It has been found that when there are high levels of gamma waves in the brain, just as when we laugh in a sustained manner, we experience a greater increase in memory, an improvement of the sensory perception and of the attention span, an increased speed of data processing, and a state of complete compassion and happiness. For this reason, one of the key features of my training is to convey to the participants the power of unconditional laughter and subsequently to guide them to live the moment of yoga nidra, as they call it in India.

Yoga nidra is a set of thousand-year-old yogic practices that promote a complete physical, mental, and emotional relaxation while the state of consciousness remains suspended between wakefulness and deep sleep in a hypnagogic state. During this kind of experience, the alpha waves of the brain are prolonged, while the mind becomes considerably more receptive. It was observed that fifteen minutes of deep relaxation is the equivalent of a couple of hours of restful sleep, which is why this practice is especially recommended to those who suffer from insomnia, in addition to be considered a valid aid against psychosomatic illness and an excellent remedy for musculoskeletal tensions. Even today the Oriental Masters during yoga nidra consciously withdraw their mental attention from the objective world to access another reality, the inner one, varying their state of consciousness and becoming more intuitive to access the sources of creativity, artistic expression, and deeper knowledge.

"TEN YEARS FROM NOW YOU'LL LAUGH AT WHATEVER IS STRESSING YOU OUT TODAY. SO WHY NOT LAUGH NOW?"
—*Tony Robbins*

Every human being experiences in his own life the need to let go and break free from those repressed emotions that when they are withheld and are not processed often cause restlessness and discomfort of various kinds and severity, even at the physical level.

According to science, in general emotions produce a quantity of hormonal changes. The stressful ones, for example, increase the secretion of adrenaline and noradrenaline, of adrenocorticotropin hormone (ACTH), of cortisol, of thyroid hormone and growth hormone as well as inhibiting the secretion of insulin, testosterone, and estrone.

In these years of experience with thousands of people I have observed that the practice of laughter causes a profound positive change, which is gradual and creates an improvement in the lives of those who practice it, precisely because it acts at the emotional level. Unconditional laughter should be considered a proper supplemental therapy to traditional medical and pharmacological treatments, given the well-being it brings us, since the primary aim of any therapy is to improve the state of physical and mental health of those who use it.

It is extraordinary that in a short time the practice of unconditional laughter techniques can reconnect us to our most intimate parts, our wiser and more spiritual self. More than any other discipline this can restore our vital energy, which is one of joy.

It's necessary to cultivate an attitude of being happy by engaging every day, from the early morning when we awake, in pleasant routines that promote our well-being and a good mood.

Teaching and promoting "the daily practices of happiness" has allowed me, for one, to practice them, to test them and to see what huge benefits they bring in the various areas of life: from the familial to the professional, from the relational to the individual. If it is necessary to promote our physical well-being by training ourselves on a weekly basis—by attending yoga classes or running or cycling for miles—in the same way we need to take care of our inner well-being and wisely cultivate the beauty of our inner self by simple gestures of genuine gratitude toward ourselves.

⁓ ⁓

"GETTING UP IN THE MORNING,
SMILE TO YOUR HEART, YOUR STOMACH, YOUR LUNGS, YOUR LIVER.
AFTER ALL, A LOT DEPENDS ON THEM."
—*Thich Nhat Hanh*

⁓ ⁓

Instead of always looking outward at all those horrors the daily newspapers and television continually expose us to, it is necessary to focus on everything that can arouse in us emotions, sensations, and feelings of peace, beauty, and harmony. Unfortunately we do not realize how much influence the outside world has on our life, on our way of thinking, of acting, and therefore of being.

We get used to thinking the same way other people think, acting as if we have been induced with mass hysteria. Rather than realizing the beauty of our planet, we sadly become addicted to the ugliness and hatred around us and are filled with negative emotions that do nothing but destabilize our real nature.

The practice of laughter has a fundamental role in this view of reality because it allows our extraordinary inner strength to cleanse us of all the emotional toxins that stagnate in us. At least once in our lives, every one of us has experienced that extraordinary liberating feeling that follows a good laugh, perhaps in good company. In that cathartic state that arises, every discomfort disappears, if only temporarily.

Our body is not able to recognize when a laugh is spontaneously generated compared to when it is voluntarily induced through a series of exercises combined with the repetition of the mantra "ho-ho, ha-ha." In both cases the benefits are the same, which means we can laugh to unleash all the well-being that laughter can give to anyone who practices it.

For this reason, unconditional laughter has been practiced for years in institutes for the elderly, hospitals, hospices, and cancer institutes as a valuable complementary treatment to traditional medical care. Compared to other great methods that have the purpose to give relief to people, the unconditional laughter allows the "chemistry of happiness" to reach those facing the experience of illness, giving them enormous opportunity to establish the necessary balance with themselves and their own emotions.

Every year I work with many multinational companies, supporting managers and employees to teach them to manage the distress that causes a negative impact on the individual, both at a psychophysical and an emotional level, and that has inevitable repercussions on the performance of organizational structures, causing adverse effects on the operating and production cycle.

When we experience severe stress, this can degenerate to cause diseases such as chronic fatigue syndrome, general anxiety disorders, panic attacks, musculoskeletal discomfort, and impairment of the immune system, consequently increasing the chance of becoming ill more easily.

Stress always involves a negative impact both at individual and at social and collective levels, and this is one of the reasons why the companies have understood the need to remedy the spread of this insidious disease called "negative stress," allocating resources and energies for the achievement of the well-being within the organizational structures.

Spreading the laughter therapy in Italy and in the world, I understood that this methodology is not sufficient to help people to improve their lives because any change can be real and lasting only when there is a greater awareness, knowledge, and understanding of the individual self. It is correct what Roberto Assaggioli wrote in his "Saggezza sorridente" ("Smiling Wisdom") when he said: *The ancients appreciated laughter so much that they considered it a divine gift and a healthy drug. However, maybe never before have we been so much in need of this drug. Men are now tense, agitated and hectic. The mania of speed, the thirst for possessions and conquest beset, strain and wear our bodies and souls. Even without giving up everything that is dynamic, constructive and heroic in our time, we need to correct excesses, adapt and balance those extreme trends. Three things, above all, the modern man must adapt and balance, in order to become a healthy and complete man: the Art of resting, the Art of contemplation, the Art of laughter and smile.*

My commitment to Professor Biava, and to those many other friends, scientists, philosophers, and businessmen who take great interest in our initiatives, will continue with a major emphasis in the coming years of moving us toward an extraordinary goal for which we live every day: the knowledge of ourselves, achieved with the overcoming of each technique because it is beyond any methodology and is what we define as **the practice of love**.

HAPPY

"Biava's intuition contains the solution to the problem that so many researchers
all over the world have tried to solve,
the solution they've been looking for:
how to treat cells that multiply in the body
without regard to the integrity of the organism.
The relevant intuition is that there is a gentler and more effective way:
reprogramming malignant cells rather than eradicating or killing them.
With a right program they turn into normal, healthy cells,
or die naturally and spontaneously."

ERVIN LASZLO

5

THE DISCOVERY OF THE CODE OF LIFE

PIER MARIO BIAVA

"Fog in the Padana Valley."

This was a kind of leitmotif, with which the Gazzettino Padano punctually concluded the weather forecast in its radio broadcasts in the sixties of the last century. And indeed the fog was what characterized the landscape during late autumn and winter in one of the most foggy areas of the Po valley: Lomellina, in the Province of Pavia. Mists, which in my childhood and youth were very dense and for many months of the year would prevent you from seeing a single ray of sunshine. Mists enveloped everything and made you feel part of a muffled environment that protected you from vital light, enclosing you in your little reality—the square with the church, the street of the school, the hedges, the walls of the vegetable gardens and gardens with bare trees, with branches that on the coldest days were often full of frost or rime, which made the landscape look even more surreal and fantastic. That landscape can deeply affect a growing child's character, his mood, his way of relating to others and with all things: the fog that envelops everything protects you, creates a halo around you that minimizes any excessive impact of the reality that surrounds you, building a muffled barrier that covers and cushions everything. That evanescent and surreal environment actually protects you against being born. The trauma of living and confronting the things of the world is procrastinated. You feel like when you are in the womb, protected and sure that nothing will happen to you nor hurt you. However, the lack of confrontation with the trauma of existence means that your life goes by, like everything around you, in a slow and veiled way so that one grows with little desire to grapple with the skill and abilities of their own body—certainly not like the children growing up in Naples or in the southern seas, lively, in constant motion, with quick reflexes and the desire to move and do to develop their skills in the fastest way possible. Things that a child living in the mists just does not take into consideration and does not even know.

The fog protects you, but at the same time the lack of light makes you more introverted and leads you to melancholy, so that, if on the one hand you feel protected, on the other you do not feel the desire to try to break the shell that surrounds you and acts as your shield. You know you should live your life completely, because in the end you realize you have been born and are no longer in the protective maternal womb. You realize that you are passing through here and feel a sense of existence precariousness. This in turn causes a feeling of uncertainty, which is opposed by a strenuous effort to counteract the inevitable end.

The contradiction in which you live marks your existence forever and makes you reflective, prone to introspection, to asking yourself the reason for everything, to asking questions about the meaning of our being in the world and about the transience of our life. A subtle vein of melancholy shapes your character, becoming one of the basic characteristics of your personality.

Melancholy, often seen as a condition that blocks you from action and makes your life painful, can actually be an invaluable resource: it is a condition that doesn't allow you not to be in tune with yourself, with your lived most intimate experiences, with your desires and your ideals. In fact, as far as I'm concerned, I have to say that melancholy has never stopped me, it has never provoked in me detachment or passivity before the events in my existence, and has never shattered my dreams. On the contrary, it has always created a continuous push to indomitably pursue what I have always considered right to realize, my aspirations and my goals; the precariousness of existence gives you incredible stimulus to try to leave behind something that remains over time. Desolation, after all, has always been a huge creative booster to me because only in the moments in which I detach myself from the concreteness of existence and free my mind to visit unexplored horizons, the sadness melts and disappears like snow in the sun.

Thus dejection never stopped me from following what my mind always dreamed of and my heart has always suggested to me. In other words, it never permitted me to be unaware of my deepest feelings and with my most intimate experience in pursuing what I thought was right and important for me and for those around me.

After my childhood was marked by the dense fog of the Po Valley, my experience was above all shaped by the example of my parents, my mother and mainly my father, two parents with a big heart, who always tried to help others even in the most difficult situation—people who have never given importance to the fatuous things in life, to money, to appearances, but to living in harmony with others and above all never thinking about their own well-being separately from that of others. All of that gave me incredible strength and fostered a positive attitude towards the world. It surely guided me to remain at the helm even through the most difficult storms one encounters in the harsher moments of one's existence.

This led me to believe in myself and to never recede in face of difficulties when trying to realize my ideals and my dreams. Their example gave me confidence and made me grow in a serene way, so that any slight sense of veiled sadness did not compromise my openness to others. Rather, it gave me endurance and strengthened in me the will to be optimistic and keep smiling, willing to seek the most suitable and least traumatic way out of difficulties, for me and for others, at every opportunity.

Fortunately my inclination to feel melancholic has never stopped me from experiencing moments of joy and happiness. In fact, I believe that even the slightest feeling of discomfort has made my joyous moments much more intense and appreciated than those of a person who has a cheerful background. Thus, especially in adolescence when the first loves bloom and give you the enthusiasm for being able to live a full and deeply felt life, you feel the profound happiness of existence. You go to the first dates full of excitement and fears, which make your heart beat fast and make your eyes shine with tension and expectations. At the first meetings, you look for the glow in the eyes of the desired person who suddenly comes out of the fog, large and gleaming in the white mist that covers and hides everything, but then lets you see clearly what you want to find and see: the soul of your beloved.

And so, with the continuous overlapping of these different feelings and emotions, I lived in the province of Pavia up until I got my degree. Then, in one of the fundamental moments in which the destinies of one's existence are determined, a sudden rethinking of the objectives that you were set to achieve in the medical profession, you realize those objectives have changed, and so you find yourself in a completely different situation than you had envisaged. Therefore, after having spent a lot of time on biomedical research on auto-immune diseases and leukemia during my formative years at the University, rather than deciding to continue research of these pathologies, my choice had leaned towards the study of the human and psychological sciences. A change of perspective of such proportions had initially upset my life, as I have already described in a previous book entitled *Cancer and the Search for Lost Meaning* published by Springer. But in that very book I first clarified to myself, reconstructing the thread of existence, the reasons behind that strange choice, as sometimes motivations that push you in an unexpected direction seem at first irrational and absurd, but for inscrutable reasons they bring you a new and different view of reality that opens perspectives that would never have been glimpsed at following the traditional ways of biomedical research. That was what had happened to me, and after a brief period spent in Reggio Emilia, I moved to Trieste where I was offered an assistant position at the Institute of Occupational Medicine in the University of that city by Professor Ferdinando Gobbato, a very good doctor, certainly one of the most knowledgeable and well-prepared doctors that I have ever known. He had followed my studies during my specialization in that field at the University of Padua.

I believe that Trieste is one of the brightest cities on the planet. Many days in the year the sky is blue and the sunlight usually so intense and penetrating that it permeates even the narrowest streets, where one would think it would be impossible for it to get to. That light, which envelops and illuminates everything, makes you breathe more deeply and gives you a sense of well-being and energy that gives you the joy that I felt as a child only in the months of spring when nature awakens and the green of the trees and lawns together with the lush colors of flowers brings back the joy of being alive and happy to exist. Thus, the light of Trieste along with the character of the Triesteans who take life as it comes and accept with a certain fatalism whatever existence holds for each one of us, have further contributed to ensuring that from then on I was even more serene, secure, and determined to pursue what seemed to me the right thing to research and implement. In fact, in Trieste I was almost obliged to resume the research I wanted to do, but from a completely different perspective from the one I would have undertaken if I had stayed at the University of Pavia to continue my research on oncological and autoimmune diseases. In that case, the studies would have followed an obligatory and traditional path, on already beaten tracks where it would have been necessary to bring only specific precise contributions to a mechanistic framework and understanding of biology and life. It is the type of studies that to this day are done in molecular biology laboratories where research proceeds with a linear approach that unfortunately very often does not take into account the interrelations that exist at the level of complex biological structures such as living organisms. Thus, while this timely research can be very useful, if conclusions of the studies do not include interpretation from a broad vision of the complexity of the biological networks that constitute living organisms, they risk being misleading because they seem to suggest that there can be simple solutions to complex problems. It can be even worse if the research done with this reductive perspective involves genetic manipulations, whose consequences at the level of ecosystemic biological networks are often unpredictable. But we will have the opportunity to return to these issues and discuss them in a much broader and more in-depth way after the various aspects related to the different types of approach to biomedical research have been clarified.

As it was, in Trieste, upon my arrival, I soon came across a problem from which I could not escape. Despite the clear skies, I knew that there was an important risk to human health in the fresh and sparkling air of that city. In fact, among the pollutants that are the most common and best known to be usually present in the air of all medium to large cities, in Trieste there is one dangerous pollutant that could represent a much higher risk for citizens of that city than for any other. In fact, in the late seventies the port in the gulf of Trieste in the Northern town of Monfalcone was closed by the largest shipbuilding yard in Italy, and to the south the gulf was closed by the Upper Adriatic Shipyard. In the middle of the gulf, where the city of Trieste is located, the San Marco Shipyard in the center of the city that did ship renovation work was also closed. In all these yards, which in those years employed in excess of 10 thousand workers, they had made extensive use of asbestos and the workers' exposure was very high especially in the San Marco yard, where the renovation work involved the demolition of pipes, boilers and bulkheads insulated with this material. The exposure to asbestos, however, also concerned the workers of the other two yards, because in any case the insulation of pipes, boilers, and bulkheads was always done with asbestos. It used to arrive at the port of Trieste most often contained in jute sacks, which allowed the fibers of this mineral to be dispersed in the air. Occupational exposure in that period involved about 3,000 dock workers.

Moreover, at that time it was also used by Fiat Grandi Motori Trieste with over 2,000 workers. All those workers were to be considered professionally exposed to asbestos, but it was necessary to consider that a smaller scale of exposure could generally concern almost all the inhabitants of Trieste—at least those of the city center, because it was already known in those years that the exposure to asbestos fibers usually spread to a radius of about three miles from the places of production and use. This is what happened to the citizens of Casale Monferrato, and Broni, a town in the Province of Pavia, who in the years of use of asbestos could almost all be considered to have been subjected to some small exposure to this pollutant. One should note that even little exposure to asbestos is sufficient to cause pleural mesothelioma, and many cases of very small and incidental contact with the metal have been recorded in medical literature, in which the disease arose after a very long latency time, sometimes even after forty years. For example, there are known cases of pleural mesothelioma in family members of workers who took home the overalls used for work to be washed: cases of mesothelioma arising many years after the beginning of exposure to asbestos fibers that polluted the working clothes.

So, as soon as I arrived in Trieste, I went to the INAIL to request the number of pleural mesothelioma complaints. To my surprise and that of my colleagues, there was not even one complaint for this occupational disease. That seemed strange, and when discussing it with the Director of the Institute of Occupational Medicine where I worked, we hypothesized that this pathology was probably unknown to the local doctors (at that time it was well known by occupational doctors, but very little by other doctors, and the Institute of Occupational Medicine in Trieste had in fact just been opened by that very good professor from Padua, from whom I learned so many things, by another colleague and by me). At that point, it was decided we should carry out a retrospective epidemiological investigation into the archives of the United Hospitals of Trieste, reviewing all the folders of suspected cases which could have resulted from exposure to asbestos. Then, with clinical data in hand, fellow anatomo-pathologists were asked to review all the anatomic-histological diagnoses of suspected cases. The diagnosis of certainty of pleural mesothelioma can in fact be made safely only on the basis of anatomo-histological data and not on the basis of clinical data alone. In those days, there was an Institute of Pathological Anatomy in Trieste which was certainly the most efficient in Italy. In fact, out of the approximately four thousand deaths each year in the province of Trieste, the Institute of Pathological Anatomy had in its archives on average 3,900 anatomo-histological reports of deceased persons. This happened for a series of reasons I have already described in the aforementioned book.[1]

The revision of the anatomical-histological data led to the diagnosis of over one hundred cases of pleural mesothelioma, making Trieste one of the cities in Italy with the highest incidence of this pathology. The reconstruction of the work history through interviews with relatives had confirmed an occupational exposure to asbestos in over eighty percent of the cases, thus bringing out a causal relation linked to very high professional exposure (however, as previously mentioned, almost the entire population of Trieste could be considered exposed to asbestos, even if not for professional reasons). The publication of those data and their dissemination also through the media (the RAI TG1 8:00 p.m. news broadcast had interviewed me) had a notable impact. That led to the mobilization of the workers, which obtained the elimination of asbestos from shipyards, the port of Trieste, and Fiat Grandi Motori, thus freeing Trieste from asbestos fifteen years earlier than in the rest of Italy.

---

1 Pier Mario Biava *Cancer and the Search for Lost Meaning* (Springer Publisher), 17–18.

After that first research on asbestos, I continued the study on carcinogens carrying out a lot of research in leather tanning factories, very numerous in Friuli, where many substances classified as carcinogens were used, such as hexavalent chromium and many dyes used in dyeing departments. So, in all those investigations, I had to study in depth the classification and role of the many substances used in the leather tanning and dyeing sector. Fortunately, Professor Lorenzo Tomatis of Trieste had become General Manager of the IARC (International Agency on Research of Cancer) of Lyon, or of the International Agency of the WHO (World Health Organization). This agency was already, and still is considered to be, the most important agency in the world regarding the classification of environmental carcinogens. It in fact, with the help of some of the best qualified international experts in the world, it examines most of the studies published in the world on individual agents or production processes suspected of being carcinogenic. It then has the experts classify each specific agent as a certain, probable, or possible carcinogen for humans.

I had become a friend of Professor Tomatis. When he was appointed Director of that Agency, aware of my interest in the study of carcinogens, he sent me as a gift all the monographs published by the IARC by then: about forty volumes (more recently, up to January 2017, there were already one hundred and seventeen). After reading them, some data emerging from the reported research struck me in particular. This data was related to the different effects that carcinogens had during pregnancy. In fact, all the various research papers reported that the carcinogens, administered in the period in which all the organs and apparatuses (organogenesis) are formed, which coincides with the differentiation into different types of stem cells and tissues, were never able to induce tumors in the offspring, but led instead to malformations or abortions. However, as soon as the period of organogenesis ended, the administration of these substances induced tumors in the offspring.

The question I then asked myself was: Why is it that during organogenesis when malformed tissues from carcinogens occur but still consist of differentiated cells that stop modifying or lead to spontaneous abortions (and therefore the death of all embryo cells) but never form tumors in the mother, while tumors are indeed induced in the offspring after the period of organogenesis? Finding the answer to that question in the eightieth decade of the last century was not easy. However, after two or three days in which my mind could not stop trying to answer that question, I finally and unexpectedly came to this sudden intuitive idea: the moment the egg is fertilized, starting the process that originates life, what we could define as the code that organizes life had to be turned on and activated. Concretely this meant that during organogenesis or, as already mentioned, during the period in which all the types of stem cells are differentiated to eventuallly give rise to all the cells of our organs and tissues, a program had to come into operation, a regulation program able to modulate the activity of various genes encoding the various proteins that make up the different cells of an entire organism. This code also needed to be able to correct errors (mutations or other alterations) that can occur in different genes during the period of embryonic differentiation. Whenever the errors were too numerous, they could not all be corrected. Then, if they were compatible with life, they were tolerated and thus we would witness the birth of an individual with one or more malformations.

If, on the other hand, the errors were too serious and irreparable, then, rather than allowing the product of conception to give rise to a tumor, the embryonic correction and control system activated the programmed cell-death genes, so that all the cells of the embryo were induced to die (abortion). This was the explanation I had mentally given myself. A consequence that was to follow such an explanation had to be that in the fetus (this is how the product of conception is defined when the organogenesis is over), considering that it is possible to induce the alterations that will then give rise to tumors in childhood, the code that originates and organizes life should no longer be so efficient in correcting errors as when stem cells are directed towards their complete differentiation in the embryo. In fact, after this period in which the development of all the organs and apparatuses has been completed, the correction system no longer has the need to be so efficient. The correction processes go on, not only during fetal life, but also subsequently even in the life of an adult organism; otherwise various types of diseases, especially tumoral diseases, would be much more frequent than they already are. Therefore, these correction processes do not need to be as active and efficient as in the embryo. Once they are depleted in an adult organism, they give rise to various types of diseases and especially to tumors. Obviously, these were all hypotheses that needed to be proven. Thus the first experiments were carried out, taking the substances present in the embryo exactly in the moments in which the different types of stem cells differed. These experiments gave very positive results and the first work on this topic was published in an important journal, *Cancer Letter,* Volume 41 Issue 3 1988.

Right from the introduction of that first work it was clearly written that it had been done with the aim of demonstrating that cancer cells are cells that in the embryonic micro-environment are able to turn back to normal behavior and, therefore, tumors are reversible diseases. I believed that such a hypothesis, accepted by the magazine and partly demonstrated, would be of great interest to the scientific community.

But, unfortunately, I was wrong. At that time the idea that there was a code that regulated DNA, that is, that there was a code on DNA that could turn on or off the activity of the different genes that preside over and control protein synthesis, was considered heretical by most of the scientific world and therefore not worthy of consideration. And so, from that moment on, and for many years, I had to face a very difficult situation, in the best possible way I kept trying to carry out the research that I had decided I would never abandon. Since I was a child, as I described above, I had been taught to not renounce my dreams and certainly I would not abandon now for any reason in the world a search that had opened unexpected horizons to me and that in any case would be for me a more fascinating journey than a trip around the world or a trip to the moon. It would be a search made mostly in solitude, but for this reason even more fascinating and stimulating.

HAPPY

"We cannot solve
our problems
with the same thinking
we used when we created them."

ALBERT EINSTEN

6

OBSTACLES AS OPPORTUNITIES

PIER MARIO BIAVA

At the end of the 1980s and throughout the 1990s a great hope and a real euphoria was fostered in the research concerning the sequencing of the whole genetic code, or in the research with the aim to identify all the genes that are responsible for the synthesis of the different proteins. This euphoria was fueled by the whole world of scientific research, by all the pharmaceutical and biotechnology companies, and by the media world. Not a day went by without the announcement of an extraordinary discovery of a gene that had an important role in the genesis of tumor diseases in scientific journals and in the media world, but never announcing that this would have allowed us to find important therapies in the fight against these diseases. The image of the double helix of DNA was perhaps the most important icon of the last century. This was also the result of the substantial investments and enormous funding granted to the genome project or to the grandiose enterprise of sequencing the whole DNA.

Thus, throughout the nineties of the last century there was a real race against time among public institutions in many parts of the world and in private companies, above all the bio-technological ones, to be the first to sequence the genome. Finally, at the beginning of this century all the DNA was sequenced, and the competition between public institutions and private companies eventually had the public institutions as winners. This has been good for all of us because in this way at least the property of the genome has not fallen into the hands of the private industry but has remained a public good, so that all information is in the public domain and under the control of the community. Until the beginning of the present century, i.e., until the sequencing of the genetic code was completed, no one showed an interest in the code capable of regulating gene expression, or able to activate or switch off the activity of the different genes that are ultimately responsible for the synthesis of different proteins. Therefore during the 1990s and the first years of this century I had to carry out research on the regulation of DNA gene expression with minimal resources.

At first, in my view, that seemed to be a limit which would have given me very little chance of doing something good. But it actually turned out to be an opportunity and an unexpected resource. In fact, if I had had sufficient financial resources to do the research I wanted to do, I would have embarked on a series of experiments based on a vision of science that had been inculcated in my mind since my university time and still prevails today for most researchers. I would have tried to conduct very precise experiments, evaluating the activity of single molecules and their individual action mechanisms. After all, like all my medical and biologist colleagues, I had received very limited traditional scientific training—based on viewing life to be the result of an infinitely long series of causally linked events, a series of chemical reactions that occur between molecules as they interact and hit each other like billiard balls.

Life in reality is not at all organized this way, and later we will be able to understand the constraints of this limiting vision. Fortunately, this path of research, which would have required very relevant resources at that time, would not have been possible for me to take, I would have lost myself in the depths of a situation of incredible complexity, and I would not have discovered anything important. It would have been like looking for a needle in a haystack.

But for reasons we cannot understand, the difficulties often prevent us from making mistakes and stimulate and encourage us to find different and alternative paths. And that is exactly what I did. In the face of insurmountable obstacles that prevented me from pursuing a very traditional line of research, I looked for alternative routes and ways to get around them. And then, having to study the processes that in the embryo are responsible for the differentiation of all cells, starting from a single totipotent stem cell (the fertilized egg), I started trying to visualize in my mind the biochemical processes that were at the base of the various steps that give rise to different types of stem cells.

So I tried to understand what could happen in the initial stage of differentiation when three types of pluripotent stem cells derive from a totipotent stem cell (that is able to give rise to a new being through various stages). Those are called ectoderm, endoderm, and mesoderm and are no longer able to give rise to a new being, but only to different types of tissues. Well, what was immediately clear in my mind was that in order to give rise to three daughter cells that differ from each other and from the mother cell for many different characteristics, they must have been regulated differently, i.e., numerous genes must have been activated or deactivated in different ways. These had given rise to many different proteins and therefore to very different cells. This meant that each stage of cellular differentiation had to consist of a specific, selective regulation, which involved a kind of quantum leap responsible for a radical change of gene expression. This way, the different daughter cells would acquire new characteristics, which would make them different from one another. This was what would happen in each differentiation stage up to the final stage when cellular differentiation would be completed by forming all different tissues, organs, and systems to become the complete formation of a new being.

In other words, each stage of differentiation, based on what I had been able to deduce and visualize mentally, had to consist in the transfer of packages of precise instructions from the mother cells to the daughter cells, which consistently changed the programs of cellular development, consequently modifying the characteristics and fundamental functions of the cells that become more and more differentiated. If this hypothesis had been correct, at that point I should have turned my attention and my studies to scientific paradigms different from the prevailing reductionism. Particularly, I should have turned my studies towards the systemic-cybernetic approach and the theory of complexity. I must say that fortunately

I had a mind that was ready, and I was already used to thinking in terms of complexity. In fact, in 1981 I had already written and published a book entitled *The Hidden Aggression—Limits of Exposure to Health Care Risks* with the Feltrinelli Publishing House in the series Medicina e Potere, which was a book on complexity. In that book I wanted to show that the threshold of exposure to various toxic substances that pollute the environment, threshold values that are still used today to assess the danger of a work environment or air pollution, water, etc. have no validity from the current scientific point of view. They are intended to be believed today but are outmoded technical values adopted to limit damage to health as much as possible. Certainly, however, these limits are no guarantee that we will not get sick. In fact, in that book I had shown that the most common diseases, namely cardiovascular, tumor, neurodegenerative, bronco-pulmonary diseases, etc., or the most frequent diseases within the populations of Western countries, are the result of a subtle and hidden aggression to our health by various environmental toxic substances. In order to do this I had to demonstrate the scientific inconsistency of a simplistic model to assess how dangerous a substance is in causing damage to our health. This reductive model assesses the danger of a substance by studying it in isolation. In this model, any toxic or dangerous substance is evaluated only with regard to itself as far as the damage it can cause to human health. Thus, an exposure threshold is established below what would be harmful to human health. This model, which claims to be scientifically valid, is shattered if it is subjected to critical analysis or if the toxicants in question, whose safety is to be assessed, are seen and analyzed in the complexity of a real situation. And that is what I did when I wrote that book. In fact, this book illustrated all the effects of summation and enhancement of the toxic action in a multifactorial exposure, which is the situation that usually occurs in reality. The effects of summation and potentiating were analyzed, not only in the simultaneous exposure to two or more toxic substances, but also in the simultaneous exposure to toxic substances and physical agents (for example the mere exposure to noise, not to mention the most serious effects due to exposure to electromagnetic or ionizing radiation, which often causes the enhancement of the action of various toxic substances. This is a little-known concept that is not usually considered but important to bear in mind.

Furthermore, in that book I also considered the toxicity-enhancing effects of different substances in people who take medication, or in people subjected to environmental stresses. And to finalize, I had considered the effects due to the strengthening of a toxic substance in relation to the pace of work and the work organization model. Therefore, the overall analysis of the resulting effect following the multifactorial exposure to multiple substances was also used to interpret the so-called induced injury, or the injury a worker most easily sustains when exposed to more toxic substances, stressful work, and effects of medication or physical agents. The result of such a complex analysis served to come to conclusions that the reductionist scientific model, still used today to assess the dangerousness of a substance to human health, actually protects us only from the acute toxicity of that substance, but despite taking into account the susceptibility of different individuals, it does not protect us at all from chronic and long-term effects. It does not protect us at all from the onset of chronic degenerative diseases and tumors (these conclusions, which today seem obvious, were not at all obvious in 1981, the year of publication of the book, but it was deliberately glossed over, even though at the time, I believe, those were no trivial conclusions).

Therefore, with a mind well prepared to apply the theory of complexity to the field of study of complex adaptive systems, I had begun to establish relationships with several members of the Santa Fe Institute of Complexity in the USA. This is one of the most important centers of studies on complexity in the world. Founded in 1984, the center's researchers from various disciplines do research on complex adaptive systems in a trans disciplinary way and have the ability to adapt and change according to the learning derived from this experience. Some of the main topics of study of this institute are the nonlinearity of complex systems, emergent behavior, chaos, self-organization and eco-organization. It is worth noting that the object of study by many researchers of that Center concerns the behavior of complex adaptive systems, systems which consist of a network of elements that operate in parallel, have different levels of organization, are continually under review and in check, have an implicit prediction intrinsic to the their structure, are in continuous transition, and are characterized by continually emerging innovations. In short, a complex adaptive system can be defined as a system capable of learning from experience, generating new complex adaptive systems, perceiving information as a data stream, coding it, and expressing it as a schema. So, in the late 1990s and the first years of this century I organized some conferences in Milan with several scholars from the Santa Fe Institute.

One of those conferences was attended by the Nobel Prize Winner in Physics for the Murray Gell-Mann quark theory. With him and other scholars of Santa Fe, I then wrote and edited a book published by Bruno Mondadori in 2002, entitled *Complexity and Biology: Cancer as a Pathology of Communication*.

So, from the study of the themes on complexity and based on the research that I had undertaken in collaboration with various University Institutes, including the Institute of Experimental Oncology at the University La Sapienza of Rome, with the University of Trieste where I continued to teach Occupational Medicine, and later on with the University of Bologna, and notably with the Institute of Molecular Biology directed by Carlo Ventura, and most recently with the University of Pisa, I was able to publish many papers on my research. Several appeared in the *Journal of Tumor Marker Oncology* whose publisher was John Klavins, Professor at the Albert Einstein College of Medicine in New York. In the editorial committee of that magazine there were well-known oncologists, such as Umberto Veronesi, Henry T. Lynch, the discoverer of the family syndrome that bears his name and is characterized by a series of alterations that predispose to getting colon cancer, Morton K. Schwartz, of the Memorial Sloan Kettering Cancer Center in New York, one of the most important cancer centers in the world, Professor Stewart Sell, director of the "Stem Cell

Review" and author of important publications on liver stem cells, etc., I was also a member of the Editorial Committee because Professor Klavins, with whom I had become friends was very favorably impressed by my publication of 1997 showing that the factors of differentiation of stem cells taken from the embryo of Zebrafish, chosen as a model for the study of cell differentiation, were able to activate the p53 oncorepressor gene, which was able to block the growth of various types of tumors (precisely in that year the p53 oncorepressor was considered as one of the fundamental genes for the control of tumor growth).

Although the *Journal of Tumor Marker Oncology* is published by an editorial committee composed of renowned oncologists and indexed by Science Citation Index, Index to Scientific Reviews, Research Alert, Current Contents/Life Science, Scisearch@online database, etc., it was not indexed in PubMed, so my many publications in that magazine (as other magazines did not accept articles like mine, considered heretical since they illustrated, as already mentioned, the role of a DNA regulation code then considered a hypothesis of pure fantasy) are not found on Medline/PubMed and therefore seem inexistent to most researchers, as they usually search for articles in PubMed alone.

In fact, many articles that already amply illustrated the functions of the DNA regulation code are found in detail in the *Journal of Tumor Marker Oncology* which in 2002 published a special monographic issue, composed only of articles written by me and by my collaborators, in which I had, among other things, published an article entitled "Cancer and Cell Differentiation: A Model to Explain Malignancy." In that article I presented a model of cancer that is still considered valid and in which I explained how and why the various types of cancer are formed. According to the article, tumor diseases stopped being obscure diseases whose fundamental alterations are not understood: the mechanisms that lead to cancer were clear and all the different processes leading to different tumor diseases were sufficiently explained. The model explained how cancer cells were actually cancer stem cells, i.e., cells not completely differentiated, whose alterations did not allow them to complete their development and completely differentiate themselves. In those cells the programs of multiplication and differentiation were decoupled, which implicated their continuous multiplication and consequently their aggressiveness.

An interpretation of cancer on this basis allowed one to conceive new therapeutic approaches, especially in the field of cell differentiation and reprogramming therapies aimed at educating cancer cells to evolve towards normal development. In practice, what was claimed was that tumoral diseases are reversible diseases, which means that they can revert to a normal phenotype. These ideas, until then considered completely wrong, began to emerge at the beginning of the century when DNA sequencing was finalized. To celebrate the event, a great ceremony took place in presence of Bill Clinton, President of the United States of America at the time. In his speech during the ceremony Clinton pompously defined it as a historical event because we had understood the language of God.

I remember precisely that the moment I heard those words I thought that instead we would understand at last that the genetic code did not represent the language of God at all, but that we would still have to do a lot of research before we could really understand how to form and organize life. In fact, after the sequencing of the genetic code, there was a moment of disorientation and confusion on the part of most researchers, because it was understood that DNA alone could do absolutely nothing if it was not programmed somehow.

Then the hypothesis of the existence of a code able to control gene expression emerged with acclaim, named by the scientists who hold the power and determine the directions of scientific research as the Epigenetic Code—the code that I had been studying for several years. The ostracism towards research which up to that moment had been considered heretical and therefore unworthy of any attention was finally over. At that point, my research papers began to receive respect as the result of advanced scientific research in the new century. My ostracism was over, and suddenly important magazines, which before would never have published my scientific work, started asking me not only for single articles, but whole special issues of magazines edited by me as Guest Editor. This new sign of openness and accreditation for my work at a scientific level is especially true with regard to basic research where researchers are essentially interested in emerging research, which opens up new perspectives previously not even thought of nor foreseen. Therefore, in this case, the line of research opened up by the research that I have carried out since the 1980s, is particularly interesting and much followed by several researchers. The same is not true, however, at the clinical level, where in medicine and in pharmacology the old reductionist paradigm still prevails. It has dominated until now all the research carried out by the pharmaceutical industry, which has heavily conditioned the process for the registration of drugs by the Ministries of Health of almost all the countries in the world. This is a very important topic that is worth taking a closer look at later.

Anyway, things are slowly changing even at this level. The need to find new therapeutic approaches that are not limited to the destructive treatments that are still prevalent at the clinical level is also emerging in the community of clinical oncologists.

In fact, it should be noted that at the Conference organized in Milan in July 2017 by the Italian Society of Medical Oncology (SIOM)—the official organ of clinical oncologists—a document was presented concerning my research and the non-pharmacological treatments I developed and implemented with biological substances aimed at "teaching" cancer cells to behave in a non-aggressive and destructive manner. This document, called "Position Paper," signed by pharmacologists and oncologists belonging to SIOM, takes stock of my research and in the end, it expresses a positive judgment on their part, hoping for further studies in the future. This document reports on the biological treatments I developed, in which very important results are reported in 179 cases of hepatocarcinoma (primary liver cancer) in an advanced intermediate stage, when other therapeutic treatments were no longer possible (thermoablation, chemo-embolization, systemic treatments etc.). In these patients 19.8% of cases of regression and 16% of cases of non-progression (stabilization) of the disease were recorded. All these cases 36 months later showed a significantly higher survival rate in those who responded to therapy than in other cases.

Moreover, what has proved important is the fact that the treatments I have developed greatly enhance traditional pharmacological therapies of established efficacy, namely chemotherapy and other therapies such as those that use monoclonal antibodies. For deontological reasons, I have never told any cancer patients who have turned to me to suspend the drug therapies they were taking. I must point out that to the patients who presented an early stage of illness I have always said that they should only undergo traditional therapies of established efficacy and that I wished them to recover completely. I have always made myself available to see them again in the future, but only if they really needed it. I have also always refused to treat patients with the treatments I have conceived when the oncological pathologies can very effectively be treated with chemotherapy, such as leukemia, lymphoma, multiple myeloma, etc.

So, ultimately, the treatment with biological substances derived from Zebrafish eggs (which are more than 90% the same as the human species) concerned patients in advanced stages of disease who still used chemotherapy, or in the almost terminal phase when such therapy had been abandoned because it was no longer effective. As I previously mentioned, I have never told any patient to suspend the treatments prescribed by traditional oncologists. This is important because, as you will be able to understand better later, oncological diseases are complex diseases requiring the necessity to intervene with multiple treatments in the attempt to keep them under control. Psychological support is also very important, and we will later see that they often fundamentally determine the progress of such illnesses.

HAPPY

"The world is not a mechanical aggregate of separate and separable parts, but an organic unity, a hierarchy in which the whole is nestled in the whole, or a hierarchy of holons to use the term suggested by the philosopher and writer Arthur Koestler."

ERVIN LASZLO

7

THE EPIGENETIC CODE AND ITS FANTASTIC FUNCTIONS

PIER MARIO BIAVA

The obstacles I had encountered when conducting research had not only prevented me from going down paths that at the time would not have led to any significant study. They had given me another great opportunity I had immediately taken when I grasped its enormous relevance. The studies I had undertaken on the functioning of the epigenetic code allowed me to understand that what was being studied was actually the code of regulation of gene expression, which is present in its totality and with all its various functions at the moment life takes shape. In fact, this code, although subdivided and divided into different stages of differentiation, could still be studied and understood in its global operation.

In fact, when all the substances present in all the different stages of differentiation were obtained, we would have the entire epigenetic code available, or the code capable of regulating all the genes of all the cells that constitute a whole organism. In other words, we would have had the entire code that governs living: the "Code of

Life." This possibility of studying the epigenetic code in its entirety exists only in the embryo and only in the period in which all the organs and systems differ. At that time, starting from a single toti-potent stem cell (the fertilized egg), through different stages all the types of stem cells are differentiated: pluripotent, multipotent, oligopotent, cells undergoing definitive differentiation, and finally completely differentiated cells. Once the organogenesis is over, it is no longer possible to study the epigenetic code in its entirety and in its different functions. In fact, when the organogenesis is finished, the epigenetic code is subdivided into various organs and tissues, and there is that part of the code in each organ that serves to control and regulate the gene expression of the cells of that specific organ; but there is no longer the possibility of studying all the different and incredible functions of the "Code of Life." So only when I had decided to study the code of epigenetic regulation, or the period of differentiation of the various organs and systems, it became possible to study all the different and incredible regulatory abilities of this code. And that is what I did, first of all choosing an embryo that was a model for studying cell differentiation.

The most used embryos as models of study of differentiation are:

1. Drosophila Melanogaster, or the fruit fly
2. Cenorabditis Elegans, a nematode worm
3. Xenopus Laevis, or the frog
4. Brachidanio Rerio, better known as Zebrafish, a tropical zebra fish that lives in fresh water in tropical countries

It was the Zebrafish embryo that was chosen for conducting research on all the work on the study of the genetic code that originates and organizes life for a variety of reasons:

1. the Zebrafish is an organism closer to man from the phylogenetic point of view (it has more than 90% of proteins that are the same as the human species)
2. it is easy to breed
3. it is easy to study and identify the moment of fertilization and therefore
4. identify the various stages of post-fertilization cellular differentiation

THE DIFFERENT FUNCTIONS AND THE INCREDIBLE REGULATORY ACTIVITIES OF THE CODE THAT ORGANIZES LIFE: THE EPIGENETIC CODE

The study of the entire epigenetic code and its functions has led us to fantastic discoveries. These different functions are briefly described here only to illustrate what great opportunities the study of the code of life offers.

The various regulatory activities of the epigenetic code are listed below:

1. **Anti-Aging activity**

A fraction of the epigenetic code has been identified, which for the **first time in the world** has proved to be able to naturally maintain, without genetic manipulation, stem genes **able to prevent cellular aging**. These are the same genes that Shinya Yamanaka—Nobel Prize Winner in 2012—had artificially introduced into a differentiated cell by means of a retrovirus. Such genes modify cellular cyclicity and maintain the cell in a phase of continuous multiplication but cannot be used without risks precisely because of the undergone manipulations. In our research, however, the **cells increase their life span without undergoing manipulation,** precisely on the basis of a **physiological regulation** of stem genes. In fact, if the administration of these factors is suspended, the cells return to the aging process, thus demonstrating that they have not lost their cyclicality and their normal physiology. The increase in cellular life span is due to the impedance of telomere cutting that is the terminal part of the chromosome composed of repeated DNA sequences; the function of telomeres is to protect the terminations of chromosomes, allow cell division, and protect against aging and cancer. The telomere prevents the progressive degradation of chromosomes with the risk of loss of genetic information: the telomeres act as a sort of biological clock that is linked to a maximum number of DNA replications, at the end of this the cell becomes too old to be kept alive. Then it takes the path of programmed cell death and thus ends its life cycle. The factors isolated in our studies not only prevent the cutting of telomeres, thus lengthening the life span of the cell, but also activate other genes, such as

Bmi-1 that induce the synthesis of various proteins, which prevent cellular senescence. So these factors, which can only be obtained in specific and well-defined moments of stem cell differentiation, not only increase life span, but keep cells young, preventing them from aging. This is very important because if we only lengthen the life span, but the cells age, we risk having old age with numerous problems and with noticeable physical decay. Fortunately, the factors isolated by us do not let the cells age and so the increase in life span can be associated with a good psychophysical condition.

At present the factors that have shown anti-aging activity have been used to prepare specific creams. These creams have proven to be very effective because they have led to a significant reduction in facial and neck wrinkles. We are now studying product formulations to be taken generally to act on the whole organism to counteract aging. These results, obtained with the isolated factors during the differentiation of specific types of stem cells, are almost impossible to obtain with artificial manipulations of the genetic code because the different genetic manipulations are not able to transfer the complete information in order to increase the duration of life and, at the same time, block cellular senescence. At this point the limits of scientific reductionism emerge even more clearly.

2. **Slowing down of the multiplication and growth of cancer cells**

The research carried out confirmed that another part of the epigenetic code is capable of slowing down cellular multiplication by differentiating the cells or inducing programmed cell death (this had already been observed in the altered multiplication processes in pathologies such as cancer or psoriasis). In such cases, in fact, the mechanisms of action we have studied can be summarized briefly as follows: the factors we isolate block the cell cycle of cancer cells, regulating genes (such as the onco-repressor p53 gene) or molecules (such as the protein of retinoblastoma), which play a fundamental role in the control of the cell cycle.

Following the blockage of the cell cycle cascades of regulators are activated within the cells, which attempt to repair the damage that is the cause of malignancy. If the damages are not too serious and can be repaired, they are actually repaired and the cells re-differentiate (in fact, after the treatment with our factors, we have seen that the markers of cell differentiation increase a lot, showing that the cancer cells become differentiated and transformed into cells with a normal phenotype; whereas if the alterations that led to the cancer are too serious and cannot be repaired, our factors then activate the programmed cell death genes and the cells die). So whether the cells die or normalize, the important thing is that they come out of the multiplication loop and stop being aggressive. From this point of view, therefore, tumor diseases can be considered reversible diseases, which can therefore be reverted to a normal phenotype—in other words, to normal behavior. Even in this case, everything happens without carrying out any genetic manipulation, but only on the basis of an epigenetic regulation of the treated cells.

3. **Normalization of the growth curves of rapidly multiplying cells as in those that cause psoriasis**

   Experiments have been carried out on epidermal cells (keratinocytes), the multiplication of which was accelerated by specific growth factors, and to which the specific differentiation factors taken from Zebrafish were simultaneously administered. It has been observed that the Zebrafish factors normalized the growth curves of the cells in increased multiplication rate, e.g., those that originate psoriasis. In clinical studies, specific creams prepared to treat psoriasis have shown a regression of the disease in eighty percent of the cases treated about a month after the start of the treatment. As we know, psoriasis is a disease that is especially exacerbated during cold seasons when various contributing factors come into play, often including causes linked to psychic alterations. Therefore the recommended treatments with the factors isolated from Zebrafish mainly in the periods of exacerbation of the disease; while a prevention activity, especially in subjects with psychological disorders, should also include some psychological treatment.

4. Activity in the Prevention of Neurodegeneration

Finally it has been shown that the completeness of the information and the redundancy of factors of the epigenetic code is able to prevent the degeneration of the nerve cells in a very significant way (this occurs because initially the redundancy of factors, i.e., of all the factors present from the beginning to the end of the differentiation process, first expands the number of stem cells and then differentiates them into specific tissue). In other words, what we have understood by conducting experiments on hippocampal cells, or rather on those brain cells that first face neuro-degeneration in Alzheimer's patients, is that if we want to prevent and stop the degeneration from occurring in these cells, we must simulate the exact program that life adopts to organize itself and realize itself. First, as mentioned above, we must administer the substances that keep the stem genes turned on, allowing the survival of the few stem cells left active in the brain of an Alzheimer's patient, thus keeping their number intact; then we have to administer the substances which are able to differentiate stem cells into specific nerve cells. So, in order to achieve this result, we must simulate exactly the process that gives rise to life and administer all the factors that are able to make cells perform the entire life process. This is an exactly opposite vision to the dominant reductionism that believes in treatment to cure complex diseases, as are all degenerative diseases, with single molecules. What is clear at this point is that it is necessary to change the vision we have of life and medicine and move toward different scientific paradigms. This is what I did when writing "Il Manifesto of the New Paradigm in Medicine" together with Professor Ervin Laszlo, signed by many doctors, psychologists, psychiatrists, etc. and which is also published in this book. With various collaborators I am now studying how the different specific molecules that make up the epigenetic code are able to repair tissues and therefore can be used in regenerative medicine, particularly in pathologies in which stem cell transplantation is required.

The so called epigenetic regulators can in fact enhance the positive effects related to stem cell transplantation and in the future replace the transplant itself, considering that it has been shown that the beneficial effects due to stem cell transplantation are not due to the transplanted cells but to the factors that they produce. Reading the publications that illustrated these results due to the transplant, I asked myself what the factors produced by transplanted stem cells were. The answer in this case was very simple: the factors produced by transplanted stem cells are the same factors that we take from the Zebrafish embryo which, as we have said before, are proteins and nucleic acids with regulatory properties, i.e., substances that we have identified one by one through in-depth analysis with mass spectrometry, showing that they are the same as those present in the human species.

Summarizing, therefore, the essential aspects and the results of the extensive research done, what has been reported above demonstrates that the research that my collaborators and I have conducted over the years, have led us to discover practically all the functions of the epigenetic code.

In fact, albeit in a concise and informative way, what is reported in this chapter highlights the importance of being able to control phenomena such as aging, with the possibility to extend the life of living beings, preventing at the same time their senescence. (This is important because it is one thing to lengthen life without preventing aging and another thing not to age during a long life.) Furthermore, it has been shown that chronic degenerative diseases, such as neurodegenerative diseases, which will increasingly affect elderly populations, can be prevented by the use of factors that are physiological and do not act with a pharmacological mechanism, causing toxic effects. Finally it has been shown that diseases that were once thought to be incurable, such as tumors, are reversible and that tumor cells are reprogrammable. Last but not least, it is possible to regenerate tissues by using specific regulation and differentiation programs.

All this was possible for three main reasons:

1. To have guessed, many years ago, the existence of a code that is above DNA (the genetic code that encodes proteins),

and that this new code, which we now call epigenetic, is able to regulate gene expression: in practice this is the program that transfers information to the genetic code, that alone can do nothing, if it is not programmed. In fact, DNA is like a computer hard drive that needs a program. So the insight that I had in the eightieth decade of the last century, which was considered heretical, has emerged as one of the fundamental discoveries of the present century. We can say that if the last century was the century of genetics (and the double helix of DNA, and in fact was the most important icon), the present century will be, as it is on the other hand recognized by the most important magazines, including *Nature*, the century of epigenetics. Studies on DNA sequencing have been fundamental, however, because they have made it possible to understand all this. At first we had hoped that after sequencing all the genes, humanity would have been able to cure any kind of disease, because yes we thought that DNA was "the language of God," as Clinton had said a little pompously at the ceremony for the celebrations of the end of the research. It was later understood that the solution had to be sought elsewhere: the Holy Grail was somewhere else. However, DNA sequencing has been important, because genetic diseases due to the alteration of a single gene (2%) can be treated with genetic engineering methods, while in multifactorial diseases, where there are multiple alterations, including multiple gene alterations, cannot be treated safely, although, as we shall see later, new discoveries on genetic editing seem to open new perspectives of treatment even of diseases in which there is an alteration of multiple genes. At the moment, however, the methods of genetic editing are not safe.

2. The second reason it was possible for me and my collaborators to discover the multiple functions of the epigenetic code, was the discovery that this code is active above all in the phase of embryonic life in which all the organs and systems are formed (organogenesis): at that stage, in fact, all the regulatory factors of gene expression are present, which are able to regulate and program all the coding genes the proteins of all the cells of an individual's entire body. Once the organogenesis is finished, it is not possible to study all the functions of the epigenetic code because when all the organs and systems have been formed this code is subdivided into the various organs, and in each organ there is that part of the epigenetic code that controls the physiology of the cells of that organ. So it is no longer possible to study all the functions of the epigenetic code in an adult organism. Therefore, it was really providential to have had the insight to do research on the epigenetic code during embryonic life, and precisely in the period of organogenesis.

3. My collaborators and I have been fortunate in that by studying how this code works, we have realized that it does not work as current science thinks, i.e., based on a reductionist model, according to which only searches for

single molecules, single receptors, single mechanisms of action, etc., important. (All Nobel prizes are still awarded only to researchers in the reductionist filed.) Instead, the code works on the basis of information programs that must be completely transferred to the cells in order to have the desired effect. In other words, what we have understood is that the scientific paradigm must be completely changed: life is based on complex, interconnected information networks, in which information travels at very high speed. We have seen that if we record all the electromagnetic waves emitted by our epigenetic regulation factors, these waves are able to produce on the treated cells the same effects as the molecules that are parts of this epigenetic code. Furthermore, Professor Carlo Ventura of the University of Bologna, with whom I have conducted the aforementioned studies, was able to record the sounds emitted by the cells with an atomic microscope (with its tip is made from a single atom). Thus, the cells talk to each other in a tightly interconnected network, transferring information immediately through molecules, electromagnetic waves, and sounds. This is a real concert: the Concert of Life.

A RADICAL CHANGE OF THE SCIENTIFIC PARADIGM

In the end, what turned out to be clear is that life is organized on the basis of information programs that, like applications, provide packages of precise instructions: these are inseparable units, which are not used if they are fragmented. This has led to a change of scientific paradigm. In fact, the research presented involved a different way of thinking and a different kind of thought that shifts the center of gravity of the vision of biology and medicine from a mechanistic paradigm, where man and the living are seen as mechanical aggregates on which one can intervene in an artificial way to change their behavior, to a systemic vision that sees the living as an information network that must be regulated in a fine and physiological way. Medicine is going to meet the change that physics has already undergone, when it moved from a mechanistic view to quantum physics and relativity.

HAPPY

"We are such stuff as dreams
are made on."

WILLIAM SHAKESPEARE

8

A NEW VISION OF MAN AND LIFE

PIER MARIO BIAVA

As we have seen, these new discoveries in the fields of biology, epigenetics, and neuroscience have led to the claim that at the basis of life there is a precise piece of information: it is the matrix of all living systems that we observe.

The new information-based paradigm implies a deep transformation in the consciousness of the relationship between man and nature, with inevitable repercussions on the medical studies and the therapeutic practice, which is profoundly destined to renew itself thanks to the evolution of this holistic vision. The new paradigm that emerges in science recognizes that the universe is not random: information is an important factor that gives shape to every part of the universe. Without the information that underlies the processes of the universe, the matter composing the universe would have been populated by incoherent particles unable to take part in the processes that gave rise to the complex systems we know, and life with all its variety of forms would not have appeared in our world.

Living systems can only appear in a highly coordinated universe, in which the laws and constants of nature are finely tuned for the emergence of coherence and complexity.

Living systems are examples of remarkable and coherent complexity. The coordination and the coherence of a living system implies the presence of precise information, which encode and rule every part, as well as the entire system as a whole.

THE INFORMATION THAT GIVES RISE TO LIFE: THE IMPLICATIONS FOR MEDICINE

A recognition of the fundamental role of information in the world of life has important implications for medical sciences. Based on what has been here stated so far, it must be recognized that life does not organize itself on principles such as linearity, causality and mechanism, but on principles such as complexity, information, coherence and analogy. Taking into account these concepts, it appears that life cannot be regulated through a breakdown of data, but through the awareness of the importance that information has in organizing life itself (meaning and synthesis).

From this it follows that every form of the living world is in a dynamic relationship with everything around it, and in a broad sense with the universe. In this way every living form presents an informative exchange with the network of the environment that surrounds it. It then becomes important to consider the ways in which man knows the world. We can say that man knows the world through his consciousness, which however is not a purely human phenomenon. According to the point of view of the in-formed universe, consciousness is present throughout the universe, but it is not present everywhere in the same way and at the same level of development. Consciousness evolves together with matter, whose most complex form we find in human beings.

At the biological and cellular level, cognition (Maturana and Varela[2]) common to all living forms has been recognized. Cognition is, in fact, the biological basis of the process of life, of which the information becomes, in addition to matter and energy, the code of signification. Man has different levels of knowledge of the world. In it, in addition to cognition, a primary consciousness has been identified which arises when cognitive processes are accompanied by a basic perceptive, sensory and emotional experience. Alongside this primary consciousness there is a further level of consciousness defined as secondary or self-consciousness which includes the ability to use symbolic images, through which we can build the system of values, beliefs, and goals. In the cognition-self-consciousness continuum, therefore, if cognition is expressed through a signs informative code, the reflective consciousness is expressed through both a signs and a symbolic-analog code.

A new model is therefore needed that sees the human person as a complex cognitive system to interpret which even the Psychoneuroendocrinoimmunology (PNEI) is no longer sufficient. The latter has been of considerable importance to clarify and understand the

---

2 Maturana H., Varela F., *Autopoiesis and Cognition*, 1980.

multiple mechanisms of adaptation and behavior of the human organism towards the environment. Nevertheless, in the light of the new discoveries in the biomedical field, the approach based on the PNEI model is no longer sufficient to interpret the complexity of the human organism, and therefore it must be integrated into the more extensive model that interprets the human being as a mind-body integrated information system. Figure 1 illustrates the new model of interpretation of the functioning of the human person, integrating in it the role of PNEI.

This model includes all the complex regulatory mechanisms of the mind-body cognitive system, that is, the regularities that lead to the development and maintenance of life. It is in fact to be emphasized, as already said, that the main feature that characterizes living systems is information: this applies to all living beings, including unicellular organisms, which are able to adapt to their environment in virtue of the information they exchange with it. For man, then, who is at the top of evolutionary complexity, information is part of a more complex cognitive system, in which cognition, consciousness, and self-consciousness are the essence of what we call life. It is therefore important to understand which mechanisms regulate the correct circulation of information and therefore the state of health in cognitive systems such as human beings. The model shown in figure 1 seeks to describe all information systems and regulation mechanisms that allow and maintain the coherence of the system.

Such regulation of information obviously depends on the structure that characterizes a cognitive system, which represents the material substrate on which the information rests. Living systems are therefore also conditioned, obviously, by their structure, but what defines them in an essential way is, as we have said, above all the information that they carry and process. Without information, the structure would only represent inert, inanimate matter. We may thus define the human person as a cognitive system in which informational-cognitive processes maintain an energy flow that nourishes and makes life possible while preserving the level of organization and efficiency of the system. In this way, the mind-body living system, as the human person is, not only keeps its own balance, but in relation to environmental stimuli of a different nature, is also able to improve its organization through learning.

Every living being, in fact, learns during their lifetime the various types of adaptation paths to the environment and, therefore, implements the organized information. Thus living systems learn how to choose which stimuli in the environment to pay attention to and, on the contrary, what stimuli to avoid in case they are able to disturb them. This means that the structural changes in living systems are cognitive acts. Regarding the human person, the scheme shown below could therefore be defined as "Cognitive-Adaptive Mind-Body System."

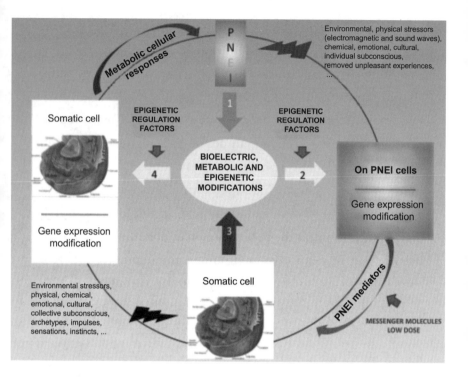

As already described in a previous publication[3] this model is reported again here, since PNEI still represents the main reference point,
even if it is outdated, to interpret the mind-body system: even
today, most doctors, in fact, adopt in this regard, the PNEI model,
although very limited and lacking. In contrast, in the model, which
is again shown here in order to spread information on this topic in
a more broad and accurate way by describing how environmental
stimuli of a physical nature, such as electromagnetic waves of all

---

3 Pier Mario Biava. Il Logos e l'Origine della Vita. Il Vivente come Sistema Cognitivo e la
Malattia come Patologia dell'Informazione. In "Il Senso Ritrovato" a cura di E. Laszlo e P. M.
Biava Springer Ed. pag. 179–201.

frequencies or stimuli of a chemical or emotional nature. Those may derive from our individual experiences, including those arising from the individual unconscious where the removed unpleasant experiences are carefully hidden, as described by Freud. Mental stimuli arising from our specific cultural vision, etc., affect the PNEI system, causing bioelectrical, metabolic, and epigenetic modifications in its cells, able to regulate gene expression and to direct the decision-making process that determines which genes should be activated and which to be deactivated. As a result of these modifications, different genes are activated leading to the synthesis of various proteins. These in turn lead to the production of the PNEI system mediators, which are well-known.

These mediators of the PNEI system act at the level of somatic cells that constitute the remaining part of the body not included in the PNEI system, on which they pour their information content. A lot of other information acts on these somatic cells that are, again, of a physical, chemical, emotional, or cultural nature. They are stimuli linked to the collective unconscious, which is that part of the unconscious evolved from the phylogenetic point of view and represented by what Jung defines as archetypes, as well as impulses, feelings, instincts, and sexual drives common to all individuals and different from the individual unconscious linked to specific personal experiences: these archetypes have great importance in determining the responses of somatic cells. The action of all the stimuli from the many sources of information cause the cells to undergo bioelectrical, metabolic, and epigenetic modifications, which cause changes in gene expression, and lead somatic cells to produce many different molecules, that in turn bear precise information that acts on the PNEI system, thus affecting once again the latter's response. Therefore, the adaptive-cognitive mind-body system works as an inseparable unit, in which information acts in a circular way, coming from the mind, reflecting itself on the body, modifying the body responses, on which, in turn, further stimuli with informative content act to produce other modifications.

All these modifications that act on somatic cells in turn influence the system to originate mental phenomena, and thus everything starts again from the beginning. The balance of an organism turns out to be a process that is continuously renewed and which is maintained by an extremely complex and coherent organization of the information that circulates continuously and instantaneously throughout the system and allows that wonderful phenomenon we call life. In the light of the previous considerations, the living organism therefore appears to be an informed cognitive system, that takes information from outside and puts it at the service of its self-organization in constant relation with the environment.

From this point of view, the disease is interpreted as an informative imbalance, and the task of medicine and doctors is to read and interpret this message, which is crucial to be able to re-inform the system and bring it back to balance. What we call "disease" is therefore to be understood as a disturbance, more or less severe, of the functioning of the human system in its relations with the internal world, with the external world, and in their mutual relations. The human system in fact constitutes a real ecosystem that interacts with larger information networks, such as the networks of the world ecosystem, social networks, cultural and information networks of all types, including the artificial networks created by man himself: it maintains its balance and health if it is in harmony with all these ecosystems. Keeping these considerations in mind, we can say that illness is an event that depends on multiple environmental factors and at the same time an event that also depends on individual responses.

So illness is both an individual and a collective event at the same time. On the basis of the consideration that all living beings are, as already mentioned and as also reported in previous publications,[4] in a dynamic relationship between them, the disease as an individual event only reflects the very limited perspective from which it is considered, while it would be more correct to say that every disease is an event that has a collective origin. Informational therapies are therefore those therapies which take account of the organism's network, of the inseparable unity of mind and body and of the man-environment system, from which a different approach can be started, aimed at identifying new therapies based on the use of natural substances that act with biological mechanisms. On this new vision of medicine, I presented with Professor Ervin Laszlo in 2013 in Stresa, "The Manifesto of the New Paradigm in Medicine," signed by various doctors, psychologists, psychiatrists, and philosophers and which is included here.

---

4 P. M. Biava, Frigoli D., Laszlo E. "Dal Segno al Simbolo. Il Manifesto del Nuovo Paradigma in Medicina." Persiani Editore 2014.

MANIFESTO OF THE NEW PARADIGM IN MEDICINE

INTRODUCTION

New discoveries in the fields of physics, biology, epigenetics, neuroscience, psychology, and psychosomatic medicine make it necessary that medical science, which so far has provided a fragmented picture of the living world, constrained through apparently independent disciplinary aspects, look for a new unifying paradigm for the various disciplines starting from what connects the physical universe to the living world, the living world to the social one, the social world to culture.

The discoveries in the world of physics lead us to argue that at the base of all that exists in the Universe, there is precise information: it is the matrix that originates the particles and all systems, including living ones, that we observe.

The new information-based paradigm implies a deep transformation in the consciousness of the relationship between Man and Nature, with inevitable repercussions on the medical studies and the therapeutic practice, which is profoundly destined to renew itself thanks to the evolution of this holistic vision.

THE PRIMACY OF INFORMATION IN THE UNIVERSE AND IN THE LIVING WORLD

The new paradigm that emerges in science recognizes that the universe is not accidental; evolution is multidimensional and is an almost universal process, and human beings, as well as other forms of life, are an integral part of it. Information is an important factor in every part of the universe. The classic idea of inert matter moving mechanically in the empty and passive space has now been superseded. The phenomena we observe are not due to mechanical aggregates of their elements but are fundamental dynamic entities intrinsically connected throughout space and time. The dynamic processes of cosmic, biological, human, and socio-cultural evolution are neither deterministic nor random: they exhibit a degree of order and coherence that suggests the presence of an underlying logic (E. Laszlo).

Understanding the nature of this logic is the perennial task of science and philosophy, as well as of religion and spirituality (Einstein observed that achieving this understanding would be as "reading the mind of God"). Without a logic that underlies the processes of the universe, space would be populated by a random influx of particles, time would not have taken part in the processes that gave rise to the complex systems we know and life would not have appeared in this world.

Living systems can only appear in a highly coordinated universe, in which the laws and constants of nature are finely tuned for the emergence of coherence and complexity. Living systems are examples of remarkable and coherent complexity. The coordination and the coherence of a living system implies the presence of precise information, which encode and rule every part, as well as the entire system as a whole.

INFORMATION IN LIVING SYSTEMS: IMPLICATIONS FOR MEDICAL SCIENCES

A recognition of the fundamental role of information in the world of life has important implications for medical sciences. Traditionally, the various specialist medical knowledge has been devoted to maintaining health as well as treating the disease.

Modern medicine is now focused primarily on treating diseases. It attempts to correct the malfunctioning of the body's cells mainly through biochemical interventions. Its remarkable achievements have prolonged life expectancy, eliminated a great deal of disease and produced many effective interventions for treatment. However, modern medicine is more skilled in treating or eliminating diseases than in ensuring that the living system remains in a state of health and well-being.

Improving health and preserving psycho-physical well-being requires a more natural and holistic approach on the part of medicine, that may be an integral part of the new paradigm that must characterize it. There is the need to take account of the flows and balances that ensure health and vitality throughout the organism, rather than focusing primarily on the causes of a malfunction of a part. A disease that emerges as a dysfunction of the cells of an organ implies a lack of information that regulates the processes of an entire organism.

However, modern medicine attempts to rebalance the vital processes in the diseased part of an organism through corrective information relating to that part, that is through the administration of compounds based on molecules, mainly of synthetic origin.

This provides an effective cure for many diseases, but in itself does not ensure the achievement of the health of the entire organism.

The limitations associated with the reductionist approach of modern medicine can be overcome. This requires, first of all, that we pay due attention to the healing and disease prevention potential related to natural substances. These substances are produced within the organism or in the surrounding environment that supports and maintains life and are the result of a long evolution that has overcome the various possibilities of causes and error.

A further way of overcoming the reductionism of modern medicine is to extend attention to the interaction between mind and body. The reality of body-mind interaction is now rediscovered by neuroscience: there is no radical separation between *psyche* and *physis* in the living system. The rediscovery of the potential to rebuild and maintain the integrity of health in the body-mind system is a result that must be an integral part of the expansion of modern medicine. The body-mind system constitutes an inseparable unity capable of perceiving and giving meaning to information and of intelligently interacting with it.

This ability to make sense of information is what we call consciousness. Consciousness is the bearer of deep-rooted values and of the rights of the living being, fundamental to give "a soul to science" and to humanize medicine in particular. The lack of this recognition is at the origin of any kind of abuse and manipulation of living beings, manipulations that may endanger the ecosystem balance. On the other hand, the interventions aimed at restoring in a natural way, without artificial manipulation, the well-being throughout the organism, are coherent with the objectives and the mission of the medical sciences. Such interventions make the use of the information governing the organism better and more complete. It is a logical development that encourages the spread of a more natural and coherent medicine with the dynamics of life.

A concrete example of informational therapy that can be associated with current medical therapies is the one that aims to reprogram and have cancer cells reverted to a normal phenotype. In cancer diseases the most serious alteration of information and communication between cells occurs. And yet even in these pathologies, where it becomes very difficult to correct informational errors, which concern both the genetic code (mutations), and the epigenetic code (errors in the switching on and off of various genes), it has been shown (P. M. Biava) that it is possible to correct these errors by providing cancer cells with the correct information. Since cancer cells are altered stem cells, it has been shown that the correct information capable of reprogramming cancer cells is carried by molecules able to differentiate normal stem cells, which have shown to be capable of having cancer cells reverted to a normal behavior. A cellular reprogramming can also be achieved through the exposure of cells to electromagnetic fields of low frequency and intensity without the use of molecules, even if of natural origin (C. Ventura).

CONCLUSIONS: NEW REQUIREMENTS FOR THE DEVELOPMENT OF MEDICAL SCIENCES

a. Need for a **new dictionary, new terminology and new definitions** of pathology.

b. Need for a **new model of the human person** based on information and consciousness that interprets the person as a complex information system for whose interpretation Psychoneuroendocrinoimmunology (PNEI) is no longer even sufficient. The complex-system thinking, able to describe the new unified reality, should recover the multidimensionality of the object-subject-environment relationship as information system-organizations and must communicate with the irrational. With this premise, the approach based on the PNEI model is no longer sufficient to interpret the complexity of the living beings and should therefore be integrated into the more extensive model that interprets the human being as an informed system or an informed psychosoma (P. M. Biava).

c. In this context **the disease will therefore be considered as an informational imbalance**. Hence the need for a new classification of diseases that takes into account the dual expressive mode of the informed psychosoma, which manifests **information according to the signs and symbolic codes** interwoven with each other. The therapist must therefore take into account the two levels of sign and symbolic language, recognize and decode them. These decoded languages represent the assumption that correct information can be returned to informed psychosoma in order to bring it back into balance.

d. Starting from this concept, it becomes necessary to create a **new profile of therapist** able to move from one logic to another **(the symbolic and the signs)**, proposing a diagnostic and intervention synthesis that takes into account these two communication modes.

e. Need for new therapies defined as **"informational"** that, based on the assumptions previously described, will enable a complex approach to the patient in which pharmacological and non-pharmacological interventions (use of biological substances), and complementary medicine can intersect and act harmoniously on the individual.

f. Need for a real and **effective trans-disciplinary integration** that cooperates on this basis.

g. Need for a **New University** capable of preparing new therapists to read the double sign and symbolic code.

From the foregoing it can be deduced that the complex epistemological background here described is in line, not only with the vision of Ervin Laszlo, but also with that of Gregory Bateson when he refers to the living being as a "connecting structure" and with the apparently simple intuition of Edgar Morin who invites us to "think as nature thinks." Being in line with these thinkers, who come from different disciplines, constitutes the best proof that the combination between the biological sphere and the anthropological one with its cognitive digital and technological extensions is the most natural, profitable and safe path to a future without risks, which instead could be very serious if we follow the path of uncontrolled genetic manipulation. In fact, if these are spread as they are expected to do in the near future, they may involve risks whose extent we cannot foresee and evaluate, both at the level of the human organism and at the level of the eco-systemic organism, that is Gaia, as Lovelock defines planet Earth.

It must in fact be remembered that biologists have been bitterly discussing for months about the so-called "genetic editing," i.e., about the technique to modify genes, of which the last one in order of appearance is very efficient in cutting off DNA errors and it is called CRISPR/Cas9 (the acronym stands for the enzyme produced by the Cas9 gene and the Clustered Regularly Interspaced Short Palindromic Repeats), that is the palindromic repetitions of foreign DNA groups, arranged at regular intervals. In practice, by greatly simplifying the problem, it is a system in which the enzyme Cas9, using an RNA as a guide, is carried out on a part of the DNA that you want to cut and modifies it, replacing it with a healthy portion. In laboratories it was immediately tested on human stem cells and on animals that are the model for the study of cancer diseases. Unfortunately, in China the system has also been used to modify germ lines, in other words, it is used for genetic modifications of fecundated ovules, inherited by their descendants.

This technique, which is not yet safe, has already shown in the embryos obtained by these genetic modifications, a number of genetic "off-target" mutations that are induced in other parts of the genome where no one wanted to intervene. Attempts to modify the germline genome mean making possible the return of policies based on the eugenics programme. Again there are terrible nightmares on the horizon, so it is desirable, as already stated by the most responsible part of the researchers, to stop the manipulations foreseen by genetic editing. The alternative to genetic editing, which is still not completely predictable as far as the results to be obtained are concerned, is the one proposed here, that is the path of epigenetic regulation of DNA. This way is much safer. It does not artificially change cells; it does not modify their normal cycle but directs their destiny where we want them to be addressed: in this way we can try to reprogram cancer cells to regenerate degenerated tissues, and to prevent serious degenerative diseases such as Alzheimer's, Parkinson's, chronic ischemic and degenerative heart diseases, etc., making stem cell transplants no longer necessary in the future.

On the other hand, with the new acquisitions in the field of information technology, large companies such as Microsoft and Google have already clearly indicated what the path of new therapies to fight against cancer could be in the future: in this case they clearly speak of reprogramming therapies of cancer cells in the ways I have been pursuing for many years and described briefly in chapters six and eight of this book. It is obviously a question of improving these results, but the path drawn is now clear and evident. It is to be hoped that it will be taken, instead of the one involving DNA manipulation, even if the latter, as it has already happened with GMOs (genetically modified organisms) is much more attractive to the large multinationals, because the gains in this case are much higher since the genetic modifications are patentable. Obviously, if the multinationals of the information, such as Google, Microsoft, Apple, etc., are also involved in this sector, then the challenge becomes open and the path to cellular reprogramming also becomes very attractive.

This is what Salvatore Iaconesi and Oriana Persico write in their book *La Cura* (Salvatore Iaconesi, Oriana Persico. La Cura. Codice Editions, 2016) on my concrete approach against cancer. Salvatore Iaconesi is a very experienced and competent computer scientist, who got cancer and wrote the book together with his wife, Oriana Persico. They contacted me during his illness, and in the book they tell their story. Moreover, they asked me to write the preface to this book, which I gladly did. It is a book to read, because it is very instructive and interesting to understand the different facets of complex diseases such as cancer.

Here is what they write:

> "Cancer cells are not reprogrammed in cancer. The information system of the body does not have or does not provide information on the direction or stopping of the replication process. In this sense we say that cancer is the loss of meaning."

In the editorial of the issue of *Current Pharmaceutical Biotechnology*[5] which is dedicated to this topic, Professor Pier Mario Biava writes: *Finally, it is important to note that research on the possibility of reprogramming normal or cancer stem cells requires an approach oriented to complexity. In fact, it requires the study of networks of substances and genes involved in the reprogramming phase, which requires expertise in a variety of different research fields, not only medical/biological, but also regarding the mathematical-computational aspects, that are required to address the complexity and non-linearity of the observed processes. We are preparing to undertake a paradigm shift, and the future will witness our confrontation with an ever increasing number of scientific studies that require trans-disciplinary skills.*

Current Pharmaceutical Biotechnology, a scientific publication of international relevance, has dedicated an entire volume to this topic, with the result of highlighting the ecosystemic features—and the tangible/intangible elements—of the scenario, as well as the need to combine approaches and disciplines to confront its complexity. In his book *Il Sensoritrovato*[6] in the chapter "The Logos and the Origin of Life," Biava continues the description of his research and its effects. He explains how those cells lost their meaning, their purpose, disconnecting from the complex

5 Pier Mario Biava, "Reprogramming of Normal and Cancer Stem Cells" in *Current Pharmaceutical Biotechnology*, 12, 2, 2001 (DOI: 10.2174/138920111794295873).

6 Pier Mario Biava ed Ervin Laszlo (a cura di), Il senso ritrovato, Springer, Milano 2011.

informational environment of the body, and how every possible solution designed to solve this problem—reprogramming these cells to find their own meaning—must go beyond the technical and technological boundaries of science and deal with society, psychology, the conscious and the unconscious, bringing them back into the equation (complex). *Medicine must restore a complex and complete vision of human beings and, therefore, the fact that human beings are not only bodies that must be treated: this means restoring the human dimension of medicine, which in its current and extreme technicality sees patients only as cases on which to implement standard therapeutic protocols.*

In this sense, cancer represents an interesting mirror of the whole contemporary society, where technical and technological trends lead to the progressive encoding of our lives, entrapping us in the data and classifications that are inflicted upon us: algorithms classify us and transform our lives, including the information and knowledge we can access and, thus, our understanding of the meanings and of our own sensitivity. In more than one way we are similar to stem cells: we reify ourselves because there are not (or we are not able to perceive) open, coherent, relevant ecosystem messages, capable of generating meaning and sense. The only way to solve this problem is to inject into the system doses of positive, coherent, essential, and significant information, openly produced by the entire ecosystem, from all points of view, on the meaning (the sense) of the ecosystem itself. On second thought, this is an interesting definition of love. So going back to the initial question: how is cancer treated? With love, and with all its consequences at a political, social, environmental, psychological, technical and technological level."

And more:

"His (Biava's) objective was not to bomb them, eliminate them or treat them as *mad* cells reduced to an irreconcilable otherness, and therefore to be alienated just as we do with mental illness. Instead he wanted to understand them and allow them to re-establish the interrupted dialogue with the other cells and the organism of which they are part, acting at the 'protocol'[7] level on the epigenetic code. His was an informational therapy based on the thought of complexity, on the systems theory, on the rejection of reductionism and violence. Or, translated into our language, a gigantic *bio-revers engeneering*[8] operation in which Basaglia, Bateson, and Guattari coexisted. The perception of this bond

---

7 The protocol is a set of rules governing data exchange activities between two entities. In computer science there are protocols for the transfer of files and network access to each level; they define the format and order of messages sent and received between network entities and the actions to be performed upon reception and/or transmission of messages or other events.

8 In computer science, reverse engineering is an analysis process aimed at the identification of the components and relationships of a software system. This technique is usually used by designers to increase the degree of knowledge of a software system when it needs to be modified. Reverse engineering techniques and tools provide the means to generate adequate code documentation; in particular, they can produce documents that have never existed or recover those that have been lost over the years. The result of this process is a set of alternative representations of the system that help the designer in the phase of maintenance and evolution of the code.

was a precise and urgent stimulus: we had to meet him. I dug Fiorello's number out of my diary to ask for help, without knowing that Pier Mario was already waiting for us: Fiorello had already contacted him presenting our case and the opportunity to follow us, but his message left on the answering machine of my cell phone, which I rarely use and that lay buried in my bag, had gone unnoticed. Pier Mario was extremely helpful from the start, providing us with invaluable, constant and sincere help, on a level that was never merely that of the medical prescription nor, even for a moment, of the scientific experiment or the clinical case. From the first phone call his voice was sweet, firm, and serene (I remember writing that it was 'soft'). Our relationship has grown and changed over time to the point that we are beginning to collaborate: a path we have just undertaken and that we do not yet know where it will lead us."

"Love and do what you will."

_____

AGOSTINO

9

LOVE: THE ENERGY THAT MOVES THE UNIVERSE

PIER MARIO BIAVA

If each of us followed the precept of Saint Augustine, "Love and do what you will," the world would be an earthly paradise. If each of us in our life, while carrying out our actions, had Love as a guide and point of reference, we not make grave mistakes; we would never hurt ourselves and others and would always be in harmony with creation and live in complete bliss. In a society where Love reigned, there would be no need of laws, courts, and prisons, because there would be no crimes, and there would be no categorical rules to follow.

If each of us followed the law of Love, we could never fear anything. If each of us followed this very simple precept in all the acts of our life, the anxiety of making mistakes would disappear in us: we would never fail with any person because we would try to help people in every way according to our possibilities, and we would never have problems with the rest of society because we would always try to follow the roads that lead to our common good. If we always had Love as the guiding star for all our behavior, the problems that now afflict the world would not be so serious and such as to endanger survival on our planet. Nowadays the dramatic situation in which the earth finds itself is due to only one cause: the lack of love. It is this lack of Love that causes people who govern the world to behave in most cases in an irresponsible way: the widespread systemic corruption that is present in all the countries of the world, is the proof of this. Furthermore, the power of finance, in an even worse way than in the world of politics, is holding an absurd speculative attitude, which cyclically causes dramatic crises in the real economy, making the sound principle of profit tied to productive investments uncertain. In fact, the globalization of the economy, together with the legislative laxity existing all over the world towards large banks and finance has enabled dangerous manoeuvres that eventually create speculative bubbles, which then burst, subjecting to great stress the actors of the real economy, i.e., in particular small and medium-sized enterprises and ordinary citizens linked to their work and to the livelihood which depends on it. Therefore, it must be admitted that at the root of all this, of the dramatic crisis in which we find ourselves today, there is essentially a cause, which can be summed up in one word: selfishness.

Today our selfishness does not allow us to see that we are doing not only harm to the whole planet and to our neighbor, but also to ourselves. In fact, each of us is part of the world: so the damage done to every living being and to the world is a damage done to ourselves. Respect for all living beings and for the world coincides with respect for ourselves and our lives: this is what our selfishness, in its narrowness and its short-sightedness, does not let us see.

Hence we need to start from here: the only way to reverse the tragic drift that drives us to the abyss is to introduce a flow of coherent and positive information into the system. And this coherent energy, which alone can change the world, is the exact opposite of selfishness and has only one name: Love. And Love has implicit in itself the concept of forgiveness.

Today, together with Love, forgiveness is the most revolutionary energy, the only one that can change ourselves and everything around us. It serves not only to understand ourselves but also to get in touch with others, avoiding attitudes that can close relationships and communication. Love and forgiveness free us from the desire of vengeance and revenge for a harm suffered. From the perspective of a higher understanding and balance, Love and forgiveness create a state of well-being because they reduce the level of stress and anxiety, freeing us from hormonal discharge caused by hatred and terribly harmful for the entire organism. In fact, hatred, anger and the desire for revenge disorganize the entire central nervous system, leading to imbalances throughout the organism, weakening, among other things, our immune system.

There are no causes of disease more insidious and difficult to cure than those linked to negative thoughts and feelings. In particular, fear and other negative feelings can change the evolution of a disease. This is an important aspect, which very often is not taken into sufficient consideration by doctors. For example, in the face of serious diseases such as cancer, when announcing to a patient his disease for the first time, doctors often paint gloomy pictures, effectively undermining the patient's hopes. In reality, no one can say how a certain disease will evolve: personally I have followed many cases of cancer patients who seemed desperate and then in fact were fine and others who seemed easy to cure, and then evolved in a very negative way.

So there are complex factors that come into play in our lives and whose scope we cannot assess. In a book I wrote a few years ago I called cancer a pathology of signification: the codes of physiological communication between cells are very significantly changed in cancer diseases. Cancer cells no longer understand the meaning of communication that comes from healthy cells in the body. Tumors are typical diseases of our time because mankind seems to have completely lost its sense, exactly as cancer cells do, which do not understand the meaning of communication that comes from the healthy part of the body. Cancer is typical of our society, because the absurd selfishness of our age makes everyone try to get as rich as possible, even if it's from dishonesty, to show off their success even if it's undeserved. The media presents absurd models for meaningful living: the need for great success, power, and money. In fact, focusing on financial success, power, and money can give us almost everything except meaning to life. The loss of meaning is what most characterizes the modern era; you can perceive it everywhere: in the unhealthy air we breathe, in the disorder and the disastrous impairment of the environment that surrounds us, which is morally and psychologically depressing, in the contaminated food we eat, in the cruel management of power aimed at protecting the interests of a few at the expense of the welfare of many, thus creating in the world a small minority of very rich and privileged people to the detriment of the vast majority of people who find it hard to live or even find themselves in a state of poverty.

In this terrible situation that creates discomfort in everyone and especially in young people, 40% of whom in many countries of the world are unemployed and therefore without any prospects of an acceptable future, we often get cancer. This happens especially to those who feel and live this lack of meaning in a more acute and painful way. If this is not taken into account, then it becomes difficult to cure the disease. I would often notice when following up on sick patients that many of them would have liked to make a radical change in their lives, a kind of rebirth that was not possible for them.

The most difficult cases to treat are those who saw in cancer the only chance to get out of a life without prospects, a life that seemed empty and meaningless. When this occurs, we need to help these people in every way to cure the disease that has affected them: the disease comes at a certain point in life because it wants to communicate something to us. It is always a signal that our deepest being sends us, that asks us for a change. This is why the medicine that only cares about the body's pains and intends to apply the best protocols to heal the body, often fails. Cancer is a complex disease, a disease in which the most serious communication errors between cells occur. To restore the lost balance, medicines or biological therapies to treat the body are not enough, but a wider intervention is needed, aimed at healing someone suffering in his soul. Diseases often come because they want to communicate us that we need to change the life we are leading, that we need to give ourselves more time to reflect and understand, to realize how we got to a situation of discomfort and malaise, and how we can fix it. Most often it is a matter of understanding that we are no longer in harmony with ourselves and with others and that we need to change our experience and relationships with other people.

It is a situation that requires an act of love and forgiveness to be resolved, first of all toward ourselves and then toward all the people who hurt us and made us suffer. It is a situation that, in order to be resolved, also needs an act of solidarity towards those who fell ill—not only an action by doctors, but by all the significant people who are part of the patient's life. It is a collective act of love that must be perceived as such by the sick person, an act of love that must envelop, protect and make him feel defended and no longer alone. This act of love helps the sick person to reactivate thoughts, feelings, and positive behavior towards the world, even in the presence of injustice and unjustifiable abuses. In this way the patient is freed from the negative feelings that suffocated and made his life sad and painful. So he can be again in harmony with himself and with the rest of the world; he can take his life back into his hands and again have feelings of love and gratitude.

This is the only way in which each of us can live in peace, in health, in harmony with all men and with creation. In this way, what Dante says at the end of the most beautiful poem in the history of humanity becomes true, the belonging of the human being, of every living being, to the rhythm of the universe, to the only movement, which has Love as its source and soul: "Love that moves the sun and other stars."

HAPPY

"Two things can save us in Life:
loving and laughing. If you have one, that's fine.
If you have both, you are invincible."

TARUN TEJPAL

10

HAPPY GENETICS

PIER MARIO BIAVA

The long journey through the discovery of the epigenetic code, its incredible regulatory abilities and how it functions as a code of meaning, making sure that communication in living beings is meaningful, has been for me, as I have already said, a lot more fascinating and adventurous than a trip around the world or a journey through space. In fact, every time I discovered something new about its abilities and functions, it was for me a wonderful surprise and a source of great joy. Whenever I happened to discover something new, it wasn't because I had done a series of logical reasoning, but because at a certain moment, while my mind was busy overcoming some difficult obstacle to the understanding of the problems I had before me, suddenly an insight made everything clear to me, and practically made me see the solution of the enigma. So I must say that I was lucky to have had to overcome so many difficulties, because every time an obstacle stopped me, to me it represented an opportunity to make a leap forward at a cognitive level, since, assuming multiple alternative ways to overcome it, in the end I would find the right solution. Now, fortunately, everyone is talking about epigenetics and many scientists are discovering that the regulation of gene expression is an event that occurs in all moments of life and that it is the basis of our ability to adapt to the environment. Everything counts and everything is important in the regulation of gene expression. Since our diet is very important, today there are specific areas of study in this field:

1. nutrigenetics, or the study of proper nutrition in relation to the genotype, which aims to identify a targeted dietary intervention for each individual, who has a particular constitution, in order to prevent the onset of diseases and

2. nutrigenomics, the study of how diet changes gene expression. For example, we know today in the field of oncology that various epidemiological investigations have shown there is a wrong diet that is responsible for the onset and progression of 30 percent of tumors, while there is a correct diet that can prevent or slow the progression of 30 percent of tumors.

Therefore the diet has an extraordinary significance in the prevention and treatment of tumors. Without going into too much detail, we can say that the diet that promotes the onset and progression of tumors is a diet rich in animal fats such as red meats, various types of salami as well as dairy products, cheese, and foods high in sugar, particularly refined sugars, and foods poor in fiber and the essential elements. On the other hand, a diet that prevents and slows down the progression of tumors is a diet low in animal fats, rich in fiber, and therefore in vegetables of all types (bearing in mind that some types of vegetables, such as potatoes should be eaten in moderation), rich in fruit (the recommended quantity is on average five portions of fruit per day). Fish, turkey, and rabbit meats are allowed, and even chicken (but only if free-range because unfortunately the breeding kind has many hormones and antibiotics that make it inadvisable). Furthermore, it would be a good idea to have three meals a day, the most complex and full in the morning, while it is recommended to have a normal meal at midday and a very moderate one, with few calories and carbohydrates in the evening. Furthermore, in-between the three meals the intake of sugars is not recommended, especially the refined kind (for example coffee with sugar) because refined sugar quickly enters the circulation and this leads to a peak of insulin in the blood, something to be avoided as insulin is a factor that promotes the progression of tumors.

Between meals only fruit intake is recommended, as fruit contains complex carbohydrates and many antitumor factors; therefore, it is allowed. There are also many natural substances that have an antitumor effect. Some are mentioned here, but for further information on the subject one should refer to specialized texts. Many food components have the potential to cause epigenetic changes in humans. For example, broccoli and other cruciferous vegetables contain isothiocyanates, while polyphenol compounds found in green tea and curcumin, a compound found in turmeric (*Curcuma longa*), can have multiple beneficial effects, modifying gene expression and thus preventing the onset of tumors. Also resveratrol, contained for example in red wine, or myo-inositol have various beneficial effects, both anti-inflammatory and anti-degenerative.

Diet is not only important for the prevention and treatment of many chronic degenerative diseases, but it is also important during pregnancy to prevent future diseases in unborn children. In fact, epidemiological studies have shown that individuals born to mothers exposed to caloric restrictions during pregnancy for various reasons have a higher rate of chronic diseases such as diabetes, cardiovascular disease, and obesity than their siblings. This appears to be related to epigenetic changes: changes in gene expression during development in the uterus may persist during adult life. Some deficiencies in pregnancy can give rise to known malformations: for instance, it is known that the deficiency of folic acid in pregnancy can be responsible for the birth of a newborn with spina bifida. Movement and exercise are also important in epigenetic regulation of DNA. For example, it has been shown that after physical exercise, chromatin changes occur in the cell nucleus, which causes the DNA to synthesize proteins that promote fat breakdown. This shows that our body and our muscles adapt plastically to what we do in our movements and the muscle exercises performed during the day.

Thus, exercise can be considered a medicine and a means to modify our epigenetic code and improve our state of health. As described in chapter eight of this book, the environment in which we live profoundly conditions our balance and our state of health according to the principles of the adaptive-cognitive mind-body model.

I want to emphasize here that it is both the external environment, the landscape that surrounds us, the air, the water, the nutrition, the social environment, and our internal environment, i.e., our sensations, emotions, our thoughts and desires, which profoundly change our epigenetic code. If this occurs in the early stages of life, epigenetic changes can have a significant influence on an individual's adult life as far as our physical and mental health. All the factors of the external environment including the climate, lack of sunshine, our human relationships, and social circumstances constantly change gene expression and lead to imprinting that sometimes lasts a lifetime.

At the beginning of this book I described how the fog and other social factors, especially related to my family and my parents, had had a profound impact on the formation of my character and how still today I am behaving according to the models I learned in my childhood and youth, including that of pursuing my dreams and not betraying my deepest feelings. What genetics has told us so far, and which in part continues to tell us, is that each one of us is the result of his genetic constitution: from his predisposition to diseases, to his intelligence, etc., everything is linked to the genetic makeup.

Genes, as we know, are parts of the DNA, which are ultimately responsible for protein synthesis and therefore determine what one is and what one will be. It is not possible change our genes, except through genetic manipulations (so scholars still claim today, who only share the reductionist paradigm of science). Therefore, one is fortunate if he has good, non-fragile genes that can keep him in a healthy state for a long time. This is true, but only partly true, because in reality much of the research of recent years has been telling us a different story. What I have been trying to tell you about cancer diseases, for example, which are still considered by most scientists and oncologists as non-reversible diseases, is actually a different story: most cancers depend on lifestyle, different environmental causes, exposure to various carcinogenic substances that can act on the genome to cause mutations, and also epigenic alterations. All these alterations, as I have tried to explain and demonstrate can be bypassed and the tumor cells can be reprogrammed, returning to being cells with a normal phenotype, using specific and targeted programs that can be found in the embryo at the moment in which life is formed.

In these last pages I have described how everything counts in the control of gene expression: the diet counts, physical exercise counts, mental and emotional states count, environmental characteristics count, family and social relationships count, and all this counts in maintaining or not our state of health and the integrity of our genes, thus preventing diseases. But when a serious illness, such as cancer, is established, then targeted treatments must also be implemented. In this case it is necessary to implement a treatment aimed at correcting more specifically the errors induced by the tumor on the genetic and epigenetic code: it is a matter of using the specific factors of the epigenetic code taken during cell differentiation, which, as we have said, are either able to repair the damage that is the cause of malignancy, reprogramming the cells and differentiating them into normal cells, or are able to induce programmed cell death (apoptosis). In both cases the result is the same:

the tumor disease can be controlled and in some cases the tumor can regress. The same is true in the presence of chronic degenerative diseases, such as neurodegenerative diseases, psoriasis or other complex diseases. Also in this case we must use the specific substances taken at different times of embryonic differentiation, or we must use the specific programs which can repair different kinds of damage. These programs are the same ones that life uses to self-organize: each of them is able to perform specific tasks and precise functions, and each of them must be used specifically to achieve the desired results. As we have said, in the presence of specific diseases we must use specific epigenetic programs. This will be the way in the future, even though for the moment all research is still focusing on genetic manipulation, and for a number of years we will still have to deal with "genetic editing," that biotechnology companies will focus on and make large investments in.

This will happen above all for economic reasons because genetic manipulations are patentable, and therefore the possible gene therapies will be in the hands of the most important multinational companies in the world, which will aim to make huge profits. There is only one hope: that the multinational companies that now govern the world of information technology come into play because they have understood that the future of science will be cellular reprogramming. This approach will not only concern cancer diseases, which in the future will be able to be tackled in an innovative way, but in general will cover all chronic degenerative diseases, metabolic diseases, inflammatory diseases, auto-immune diseases and anti-aging treatments. In fact, as I mentioned very briefly before, it is already possible to increase the duration of our life, but it is also possible to prevent aging. This is very important, because if we increase life span, without preventing aging, we eventually become like Methuselah and we will have a poor quality of life, which we will not accept willingly. But if we increase life span and prevent aging at the same time, as experimentally demonstrated and published,[9] without performing genetic manipulations, then the situation changes completely and the path becomes viable and desirable.

Therefore, as already mentioned, with the various collaborators it has been shown that the different programs that together constitute the entire epigenetic code have the multiple functions described in chapter seven. If these are the main strands that will concern the future of science, there is one thing that we can do right now in every moment of our life and that will help keep ourselves healthy: loving and laughing. The beneficial effects of love and forgiveness have already been stated. There are studies on laughter therapy and all-round yoga (so asana, pranayama, meditation, etc.) that report how these practices are able to epigenetically inhibit the genes responsible for the synthesis of proteins linked to inflammation and stress (already in 2008 a publication on Plos One reported a study on yoga and its beneficial effects on gene expression). Moreover my friend Nitamo Montecucco, who in his Center

9. P. M. Biava, Canaider S. Facchin F, Biancone E. Ljungberg L. Rotilio D. Burigana F. Ventura C., *Stem Cell Differentiation Stage Factors from Zebrafish Embryo: A Novel Strategy to Modulate the Fate of Normal and Phatological Human (Stem) Cells.* Curr. Pharm. Biotechnol, 2015; 16 (9): 782–92. Guest Editor: P. M. Biava.

"The Global Village" in Bagni di Lucca organizes many meditation and Mindfulness courses, has shown in various studies how through meditation there is an epigenetic rebalancing that leads to an increase in efficiency of the hormonal system and the immune system from activation of centers that reduce stress, so that a sense of well-being, pleasure and increased self-confidence is achieved. Then the laughter and the therapy of laughter bring this feeling of well-being and pleasure to its peak. Laughter therapy, as practiced in Richard Romagnoli Workshock, where besides an amazing laugh only he knows how to impart, a philosophy of life is presented based on love, on the acceptance of what life offers us, on forgiveness and on the sense of gratitude towards every living being and all creation. It represents a real therapy, which significantly increases the conditions of the well-being and health in each one of us.

Everyone knows that laughing is good for our health, but perhaps not everyone knows that in support of the beneficial power of laughter, numerous clinical studies have been carried out, especially in recent years, which have shown that an optimistic attitude towards sickness aids the healing process for various ailments.

Even regarding the approach to such a widespread and complex pathology as cancer, testimonies of both doctors and patients describe how the use of laughter helps patients to better face the disease and at the same time helps to instill confidence in their treatments.

The scientific study of the effects of laughter and positive emotions on human life is a relatively new field of research that has developed particularly in the healthcare sector thanks to the contribution of doctors and scholars such as Patch Adams, recognized as the founding father of "smile therapy" or Clown therapy. However, nowadays the "medicine of the smile" has gone beyond the walls of hospital wards and entered private homes and offices. Laughter is in fact used as a cure even by Coaches—and Richard Romagnoli is unsurpassed in this—to help people achieve serenity, well-being and happiness. There is now a lot of research on this. We have already discussed how epigenetic treatments can improve the conditions of the cardio-circulatory, muscular, and immune systems through the PNEI system (Psico Neuro Endocrino Immunologic). It has also been mentioned how this system, connecting the brain to the cells of the immune-competent system (cells that have the task of reacting specifically to any foreign agent), improves our defenses against multiple external aggressions.

Mind and body are not in fact two separate worlds but are two parts in continuous reciprocal influence, which act as a single cognitive network: man in his psychosomatic unity. It has long been proven that good mood and confidence strengthen the organism, while depressive states favor the onset of diseases and their aggravation. To give more detail, laughter therapy acts in depth on our state of health because it not only increases our immune defenses but also the production of many substances including serotonin and endomorphins that improve our well-being and mood. Endorphins are called the "happiness hormones" due to their ability to cause a sensation of well-being. Endorphins are neurotransmitters produced by the anterior pituitary gland, whose main effects, in addition to the sensation of well-being, are sedation of pain, vasodilatation, thanks to the release of nitric oxide in circulation, appetite regulation and intestinal and pancreatic activities. The release of these substances is linked to certain activities such as sexual activity, intense physical activity, falling in love, and techniques such as acupuncture.

ADRENALINE

Adrenaline is a neurotransmitter and a hormone secreted by the adrenal glands. Belonging to the catecholamine group, it is called a "stress hormone." In stressful situations, in fact, the secretion of this hormone increases, preparing the body for an attack or escape reaction: heart beats increase, blood vessels are reduced in size, and bronchioles are increased. In the case of laughter, as with cortisol, the production of adrenaline is reduced. This fact, combined with the action of endorphins, helps the person achieve a state of relaxation and well-being.

NATURAL KILLER CELLS (NK)

Natural killer cells are lymphocytes specialized in the recognition of non-self cells, such as infected and tumor cells. NK lymphocytes act by releasing substances that, by binding to the plasma receptors of cells considered foreign, induce programmed cell death (apoptosis). Scientific studies have shown that laughter causes an increase in the activity of natural killer cells. This increase remains up to 12 hours after stimulation, when the values still have not returned to the basal level. This fact can be very useful for the prevention of some diseases, above all, as already mentioned, tumor diseases.

The changes caused in our body by laughter therapy are not limited only to the modifications of the PNEI system mentioned above. In fact, the cells of the PNEI system in turn act on all the cells of our body, leading to epigenetic changes responsible for the regulation of various genes, which change positively the state of well-being and health of all of our cells. In turn, somatic cell changes act on the cells of the PNEI system, as evidenced in the model defined as "Mind-Body Cognitive-Adaptive System," thus closing the circle. It is therefore a therapy that acts in depth on every cell of our body, leading to changes in the expression of our genes, which has no side effects of any kind and which is good for us all in every moment of our lives. And this is why I have written this book with Richard Romagnoli, which I hope will be of help. It is worth remembering: "two things save us in life: loving and laughing. If you have one, that's fine. If you have both of them, you are invincible." And "a day without a smile is a day wasted" and this is what Richard Romagnoli teaches and transmits with incredible energy, love, and passion in his Workshocks.

HAPPY

"It is amazing how affability combined
with compassion can benefit the experienced
doctor and surgeon: it is a wonderful medicine
for long and depressing diseases,
when the fear of death often takes over,
as it consoles both the sick and their relatives
in tears, so much so that they can wait with an
almost serene spirit for whatever may happen;
and those who should encounter death or
madness are so comforted that their condition
improves, due to new hope and a positive state
of mind. Because nothing remedies the damage
nor appeases the terror of long,
painful, incurable diseases
both in the sick and their relatives
as much as a compassionate and warm talk."

LEONARDO BOTALLO

11

CHOOSE TO DISSOLVE YOUR PAIN

RICHARD ROMAGNOLI

Dad's scream on that Sunday ripped my peace of mind forever. I woke up with a start in bed, my heart beating like crazy in my throat. After that desperate scream that tormented me for many months and robbed me of my sleep, a heartbreaking cry announced the gravity of what was happening, and for the first time I saw my father in despair. The doctor, a family friend, had thought of leaving a message on the answering machine at home informing us that the furuncle that dad had on his face was something else, a malignant carcinoma.

The histological examination established the effect of a cause that science was never able to explain to us. Only in later years, thanks to the presence of my master and to my wife's love, could I dissolve the pain of the experiences I lived through and the anger for the insensitivity of that doctor. During the long period of his illness we decided, together with my family, to always stay close to Dad, to never leave him alone for a moment, sharing every precious moment together. It is love that ennobles our life and it is always love that helps us in the most difficult moments, even in those that appear dramatic. Love can really guide us, leading us away from fear and discouragement, especially when we are willing to entrust ourselves completely to its strength, to that energy that is beyond any human limit. in order to entrust ourselves to love, we need courage: that of living life with total presence.

∽〰∾ ∾〰∽

"ONE ATTAINS MERIT BY SERVING OTHERS
AND COMMITS SIN BY HURTING THEM."
—*Sathya Sai Baba*

∽〰∾ ∾〰∽

Those doctors who communicate harshly to their patients, unfortunately, do not realize that their sterile communication causes much harm to those hanging on their words because it is shown that the word is pure vibration and has a great power, that of healing at multiple levels. The insensitivity towards those who suffer, when it is ascertained, should be sufficient to remove those who clearly show through their attitude that they are not suitable to exercise the medical profession. I have never tolerated the ego and supremacy of those few professionals, which I believe to be the minority, who, wearing their white coats, show off their professional position to fill personal gaps, destabilizing with their behavior the harmony of their colleagues and team, but above all of those patients who will have to rely on their care. It is always too late to start countering the unhealthy habit of interacting superficially and paying little attention to those we meet, but the time has come to take back our humanity to ensure that our lifestyle truly represents what we are, rather than continue to alienate our presence.

It is necessary to speak with gratitude of the excellent work that is carried out every day by thousands of professionals and health-care system operators, who with great dignity, preparation, self-sacrifice, absolute dedication and passion give their time to contribute to the well-being of society.

Several years after my father's death, my mother also underwent a delicate surgery to remove a cancer. After many hours spent inside the operating theater, the surgeon pronounced the verdict: "Your mother has only have a few months to live." Fortunately, more than a decade has passed since that day and, in addition to her rapid physical recovery, she was able to see the birth of her grandchildren, Matilde and Sofia, and continues to rejoice in their growth.

What made the difference in her case to help her to defeat the disease was the positive mental attitude she had throughout the postoperative course. Her tenacity, strength, and faith prevented her from basking in pain, facing each trial with more courage and greater determination.

During the writing of this book I had the great fortune to converse countless times with Professor Mario Biava about different issues regarding disease, research, science, and spirituality, and what I learned from this great man, who has dedicated his life to scientific research, is the importance of love, empathy, and respect that cannot be lacking in the relationship of care between the patient and the doctor.

I am sure that in the years to come hospitals will change their architecture and internal organization to become real "healing temples," harmonious spaces that welcome and inspire those who are living though their personal experience called disease to find in themselves the choice to dissolve their pain and make space for the joy of living. *Happy Genetics* is a source for all those who feel they want to give their best in what they do to transform their lives wonderfully. Each of us is connected to one another, and we should not forget this, especially when we interact with those who have entrusted their lives to us, being aware that the principle that animates our existence is love.

"AWARE OF THE IMPORTANCE AND SOLEMNITY OF THE ACT I
PERFORM AND OF THE COMMITMENT I UNDERTAKE, I SWEAR:
TO EXERCISE MEDICINE IN FREEDOM AND INDEPENDENCE OF
JUDGMENT AND BEHAVIOR AVOIDING ANY UNDUE INFLUENCE;
TO PURSUE THE DEFENSE OF LIFE,
THE PROTECTION OF MAN'S PHYSICAL AND MENTAL HEALTH
AND THE RELIEF OF SUFFERING, TO WHICH I WILL INSPIRE ALL
MY PROFESSIONAL ACTS WITH RESPONSIBILITY AND CONSTANT
SCIENTIFIC, CULTURAL AND SOCIAL COMMITMENT;
TO TREAT EVERY PATIENT WITH EQUAL CARE AND COMMITMENT,
IRRESPECTIVE OF ETHNICITY, RELIGION, NATIONALITY,
SOCIAL CONDITION OR POLITICAL IDEOLOGY,
AND PROMOTING THE ELIMINATION OF ALL FORMS OF
DISCRIMINATION IN THE FIELD OF HEALTH CARE;
TO REFRAIN FROM ANY DIAGNOSTIC AND THERAPEUTIC
OVERKILL; TO PROMOTE THE THERAPEUTIC ALLIANCE WITH THE
PATIENT BASED ON TRUST AND MUTUAL INFORMATION,
RESPECTING AND SHARING THE PRINCIPLES
THAT INSPIRE THE MEDICAL ART."
—from the Professional Oath of the Order of Physicians

"LOVE ALL, SERVE ALL. HELP EVER, HURT NEVER."
—Sathya Sai Baba

ACKNOWLEDGMENTS

RICHARD ROMAGNOLI

One day Pier Mario and I were in Milan to talk about our book. Discussing this with him was a special experience, an opportunity that allowed me to become more aware of what I practice and what I love to give to people. We were wondering what title could represent our message and Sara, my wife, who was with us, suggested: "Call it Happy Genetics: From Epigenetics to Happiness." And that's how the title of the book you are holding was born.

My deepest thanks go to Sara because standing by me as a wife is a great challenge, both for being the mother of our beautiful girls and for the extraordinary ability to always take care of me. She does a delicate job before, during, and after my training, making my job a real mission. Honestly, without her, I couldn't have experienced what I wrote here. When my Master gave us the opportunity to live next to him in India my fear was addressed to Matilde and Sofia, our two daughters. I am deeply grateful to these two wonderful souls for demonstrating an understanding for my feeling that goes beyond all logic and that has a great meaning: it's called Love. Deep gratitude for all my family, for their esteem for me. I would like to thank my closest collaborators, the members of my staff and team for being the real support even in the toughest times.

To Loretta Zanuccoli, my beloved publisher for having always believed in my message and allowed me to spread it. I'll keep talking about her in the present, never in the past. To the fantastic group of Eifis Editore for the dedication and care given to all my projects. To Davide Cortesi for his great professionalism and to Elena Benvenuti who is not only my editor, but a gift for anyone who has the good fortune to collaborate with her.

To Niccolò Branca who honors me with his friendship. And then thanks to Professor Narasimhan, the Director of the Sri Sathya Sai Mobile Hospital, for giving me the opportunity to live amazing experiences in contact with the best doctors and luminaries of India, and for teaching me a lot about "Love therapy." To the doctors of Sri Sathya Sai Super Specialty Hospital in Puttaparthi, because when I was sitting next to the Master they were in the "Temple of Healing" to put his teachings into practice, serving the most needy. To my beloved Master Sri Sathya Sai Baba for inspiration, guidance and example. To all the people I met along the way because I learned a lot from each one. To all those who, understanding the Value of life, protect Mother Earth with Love.

PIER MARIO BIAVA

I would like to thank all the persons who supported my work: first of all my wife and my children, who had been infinitely patient with me when I am completely engrossed in my thoughts, learning how to overcome certain obstacles that arose from time to time during my research. Then I would like to thank all the researchers of many different Universities, including University "La Sapienza" of Rome, the University of Bologna, and the University of Trieste because it was possible with their contribution to speed up research times and arrive at important and repeatable results in truly innovative fields such as tissue regeneration, reprogramming cancer stem cells, and others. This has made it possible to develop treatments for the prevention and integrative treatments of many chronic degenerative diseases.

Last but not least, I would like to thank all those who have contributed to spreading a new scientific paradigm in medicine and life science in the first place, especially Ervin Laszlo, who I consider one of the most important living philosophers of science, with whom I have written many books that have contributed to expanding a new scientific paradigm in science.

INDEX

informational imbalance, equivalence, 123–124
interpretation, 116–117
multifactorial diseases, treatment safety (absence), 103–104
negative thoughts/feelings, impact, 135–136
neuro-degenerative diseases, prevention, 102
parental struggle, 1
self-identification, problems, 13
suffering, 24–25
treatment, medicine (focus), 120
Distress, management, 56
Divine Nature
discovery, 4
divergence, 41
Divine, understanding, 29
Doctors
attitudes/empathy, observation, 7–8
courage/compassion/love, 21
responsibility, 22
Double sign, reading, 124
Drosophila Melanogaster (fruit fly), 94
Duality, feelings, 41

Earth, balance (restoration), 48
Eastern spirituality, study, 3
Economy, globalization (problems), 134
Ecosystem balance, endangerment, 121–122
Ecosystemic biological networks, consequences, 67
Ectoderm, 79
Ego
improvement, 37
Prâjña principle, 30
Egotism, suffering, 35
Einstein, Albert, 45, 76, 119
Embryo
cells, death, 72
models, usage, 94–95
processes, study, 79
Embryonic differentiation, code errors, 72–73
Emotional relaxation, promotion, 53
Emotional well-being, protection, 37

Emotions
feelings, overlap, 65
harmonic approach, cultivation, 16
impact, 54
Empathy, 7–8
healing, language, 18–25
Endoderm, 79
Endorphins (happiness hormones), 150–151
Energies, multidimensional network, 18–19
Energy flow, informational-cognitive processes (impact), 113
Enthusiasm, restoration, 48
Environmental causes, impact, 146
Environmental toxic substances, impact, 81
Epigenetic Code, 87
change, 145
Code of Life, functions/regulatory activities, 95–105
discovery, 141
existence, 102–103
function, 93, 104–105, 141
protocol level, actions, 130
subdivisions, 94
Epigenetic regulators, impact, 101
Epigenetic treatments, impact, 150
Eros (love form), 34
Evolution
dynamic processes, order/coherence, 119
multidimensionality, 118–119
Exercise, importance, 144
Existence
happiness, feeling, 64–65
precariousness, 63
Existential nature, discovery, 13
Exposure threshold, establishment, 81–82

Faith, impact, 2–3
Falsehood, impact, 40
Fatalism, 66
Fear/discouragement, love (impact), 156
Feelings/emotions, overlap, 65

confusion, 13
enclosure, 61
Reductionist paradigm, prevalence, 88
Reductionist scientific model, 82–83
Resveratrol, benefits, 143–144
Retrovirus, usage, 96
Revenge, desire (freedom), 135
Reverse engineering, process, 130
Richard Romagnoli Workshock, 149
Ridd, Karen, 23
Righteousness, impact, 41
Robbins, Tony, 53
Romagnoli, Richard, 150, 152

Sadness, sense, 64
Saint Augustine of Hippo, 28, 131, 132
Santa Fe Institute of Complexity, 83–84
Saraswathi Hall, laughter club (opening), 9
Sathya Sai Mobile Hospital project, 7
Schwartz, Morton K., 84
Scientific paradigm, change, 105–106
Secondary consciousness, 111
Self, 15–17
    identification, question, 14–15, 28
    recognition, 15
Self-confidence, increase, 149
Self-consciousness, 111
Selfish actions, recognition, 35–36
Selfishness
    definition, 35
    narrowness/short-sightedness, 134–135
    overturning, 48
Self-love, failure, 38
Self-opinion, issues, 35
Self-organization, 116, 147
Self-reification, 129–130
Sell, Stewart, 84–85
Senescence, 102
    cellular senescence, prevention, 97
Serenity, feelings (amplification), 36
Serotonin production (increase), laughing (impact), 49–50
Shakespeare, William, 108
Skills, development, 62

Smile therapy, 150
Smiling
    impact, 51–52
    practice, importance, 23
Smiling Wisdom (Assaggioli), 57
Social factors, impact, 145
Society
    change, urgency, 48
    well-being, 157
Somatic cells
    modifications, impact, 116
    responses, determination, 115–116
Soul, science
    study, 4
    transcendence, 28
Spirit, body (connection), 28
Spiritual disciplines, success, 8
Spirituality, richness, 6
Spiritual path, following, 29–30
Spontaneous abortions, 72
Sri Sathya Sai Super Specialty Hospital, attendance, 6–7
Stem cells
    differentiation, 72–74, 79, 85, 97
    number, expansion, 100
    transplantation, 101
    types, 94
Stem genes, physiological regulation, 96
Storge (love form), 34
Stress
    experience, 56–57
    factors, 36–37
    hormone, 151
        inhibition, laughing (impact), 49
    negative stress, 57
    reduction, 149
Student intelligence (development), laughter/smiling (impact), 51–52
Substances
    anti-tumor effect, 143
    danger, reductive model (assessment), 81
    multifactorial exposure, 82
    toxicity-enhancing effects, consideration, 82–83
Suffering, alleviation, 3

ABOUT THE AUTHORS

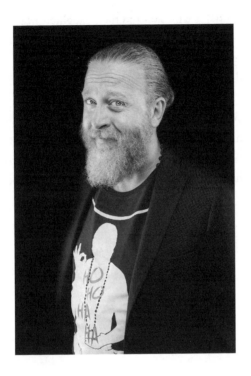

RICHARD ROMAGNOLI

Throughout his international experience, Richard Romagnoli has made a huge contribution to the spread of spiritual teachings and wellness practices with his Laughter Therapy, classes in meditation and methods of "Happy Genetics" both in Italy and many other countries. His trainings are followed by thousands of people around the world.

Richard is the author of several Italian best-selling books on spirituality, happiness, and ethical business, including the book *I Learned to Laugh*.

He created a CD of audio meditation, "Tree of Life," and produces online courses. He writes regualarly for the Huffington Post and for Arianna Huffington's Thrive Global.

He has lived with his wife Sara and their daughters Matilde and Sofia in southern India where he deepened his studies of spirituality and Hasya Yoga. He is a strategic consultant for major global corporations and multinationals for his skills and competencies in fostering well-being in organizations and increasing their production performance.

As a guest speaker at international events he has shared the stage with Deepak Chopra, Gregg Braden, Don Miguel Ruiz, Bruce Lipton. He has been invited twice to give a speech at TEDx in Italy. Richard was nominated by the international organization Stop Hunger Now to be "Global Food Security Ambassador."

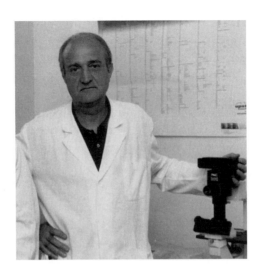

PIER MARIO BIAVA

Pier Mario Biava received his degree in medicine at the University of Pavia, before specializing first in occupational medicine at the University of Padova and later in hygiene at the University of Trieste. For several years he has studied the relationship between cancer and cell differentiation to determine the prevention and treatment of chronic degenerative diseases and the possibilities for renewal and regeneration of tissues. He has isolated the differentiation factors of stem cells that can inhibit or slow down the growth of various types of human tumors to prevent neurodegeneration and aging.

Dr. Biava has been a lecturer at the School of Occupational Medicine in Trieste for several years and currently works at the Institute of Research and Care Scientific Multimedica of Milan. He is the author of over 100 scientific papers and several books, including *The Hidden Aggression: Limits of Exposure to Health Care Risks* published by Feltrinelli, *Complexity and Biology* published by Addison, *Cancer and Research Direction Lost* published by Springer, *The Meaning Found*, edited by Ervin Laszlo and published by Springer. He contributed to "From Sign to Symbol—The Manifesto of Nuono Paradigm in Medicine" used by committees in the field of oncology and epidemiology.